*f*P

Also by Lucy Jo Palladino, PhD

Dreamers, Discoverers, and Dynamos:
How to Help the Child Who Is Bright, Bored,
and Having Problems in School

Find Your Focus Zone

An Effective New Plan to Defeat Distraction and Overload

LUCY JO PALLADINO, PhD

FREE PRESS

New York   London   Toronto   Sydney

FREE PRESS
A Division of Simon & Schuster, Inc.
1230 Avenue of the Americas
New York, NY 10020

First Free Press hardcover edition June 2007

FREE PRESS and colophon are trademarks of Simon & Schuster, Inc.

For information about special discounts for bulk purchases,
please contact Simon & Schuster Special Sales at 1-800-456-6798
or business@simonandschuster.com

Book design by Ellen R. Sasahara

Manufactured in the United States of America

1 3 5 7 9 10 8 6 4 2

Library of Congress Cataloging-in-Publication Data

Palladino, Lucy Jo.
Find your focus zone: an effective new plan to defeat
distraction and overload / by Lucy Jo Palladino.
p. cm.
Includes index.
1. Attention. I. Title.
BF321.P35 2007
153.7'33—dc22
                    2007003236

ISBN-13: 978-1-4165-3200-2
ISBN-10:   1-4165-3200-5

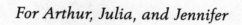

For Arthur, Julia, and Jennifer

CONTENTS

Find Your Focus Zone

INTRODUCTION

You and I live in a 24/7 culture, and someone is always upping the ante. New technology makes you more productive but pressures you to pick up the pace. You have a new cell phone? Good. Now, your boss can reach you on your day off. Wireless PDA, huh? Excellent. We'll expect e-mails, too. Mini-PC? Even better. We'll instant-message you those files. . . . Whether you work inside or outside your home, you juggle a schedule of constant demands and always-on electronics. Multitasking is rampant. For better or worse, we're rewiring our brains for what the technology industry now calls "continuous partial attention."

In the digital age of distraction, we function at new levels of stimulation and anxiety. The Internet spews information like a fire hose, but to digest information we need to sip it through a straw. Overwhelmed and overloaded, we have no time to process or reflect. Sunday is not a day of rest, but an attempt to catch up and clear your clutter. Old ways of paying attention can't keep up. We need new tools.

Attention Makes the Difference

Having control over your attention is a critical skill. I specialize in working with human attention because paying attention matters. Every one of us needs the ability to direct our attention, or we will not reach our goals. In my thirty years of practice as a clinical psychologist, I've helped thousands of people solve myriad problems by improving their attention. Learning attention management skills has made life better for just about everyone who has walked through my door, not just for those with attention deficit disorder.

This morning, for instance, my first appointment was with an executive who'd recently had a heart attack. He came to see me to learn stress management skills that will help him prevent another one. His biggest challenge is to get his mind off his highly competitive workplace when it's time for him to go home and relax. Next, I saw a woman in her thirties who is battling depression. "Everyone tells you to stay positive," she observed, "but no one tells you how." I'm going to help her unglue her attention from negative thoughts of worry, blame, and self-criticism, and focus instead on hope, trust, and self-appreciation.

I saw a college student with social anxiety who's learning to redirect his attention away from his memories of rejection and onto cues he can get from others so he can succeed in social situations. Then came a baby boomer trying to lose weight, struggling to pay more attention to fruits and vegetables than to rich sauces and pastries. A young perfectionist couple have a weekly appointment with me to practice ways to focus on each other's humanity, not on each other's faults. *Attention control* is a necessary ingredient for each of us to be healthy, happy, and successful.

How Does Digital-Age Distraction Hurt You?

When it comes to attention and the digital age, we each have different strengths and vulnerabilities. What's your style? Are you prone to attention swings, back and forth between boredom and overdrive? Or do you tend toward one end or the other—lost in space or racing against the clock with no time to spare? Take a moment to ask yourself which style describes you best.

Do You Have Attention Swings?

Most people today fluctuate between boredom and overdrive. Do you:

- ❑ Buy books that grab you at the store, but don't finish reading them at home?

❑ Buy the latest high-tech gadget, play with it while it's new, then turn it into a bookend (to hold up all those unfinished books)?

❑ Stop what you're doing to answer a cool e-mail, but have two or more half-written e-mails in your drafts folder?

❑ Agree to go to places that sound like fun when you're invited, then make up excuses when it's actually time to stop what you're doing and go?

❑ Ambitiously start a diet by buying ingredients for unusual recipes, but toss them out when they grow mold and turn into a science project in your fridge?

Are You Scattered and Spacey?

Some people find that they're more the scattered and spacey type. It's a constant challenge for them to stick with what they're doing. They spend a lot of time overextended, underpowered, and indecisive. Do you:

❑ Go to the store, browse through some books, see one you like, put off deciding whether to buy it or not, go home, wish you'd bought it, and eventually go back to the store only to find that it's no longer on the shelf?

❑ Put off buying the latest high-tech gadget, and when you finally do get it, leave it in the box until your tech-savvy neighbor comes over to set it up for you?

❑ Have six or more half-written e-mails in your drafts folder?

❑ Agree to go to places that sound like fun when you're invited, look forward to going, and then arrive late no matter what time you started to get ready?

❑ Consider starting a diet for a few weeks, go to the bookstore to find (but not buy) a diet book, read magazine articles about losing weight, and put a recipe on your refrigerator door (if there's room) to think about it awhile?

Are You Hyperfast and Hyperfocused?

Some people are wired for speed and intensity. They find it hard to say no to constant stimulation. Do you:

- ❏ Go only to bookstores that have wifi so you can stay connected while you're there?
- ❏ Be the first to own the latest high-tech gadget, trade up your current gadgets for the next generation right away, and have a gadget for every purpose?
- ❏ Check your e-mail continuously and wrt msgs ryt awy lk ths?
- ❏ Agree to go to places that sound like fun when you're invited but in the back of your mind know that if a better opportunity comes up you will call and cancel?
- ❏ If you need to lose weight, gulp down breakfast shakes and power bars—a great reason to eat on the run!

Whatever your style, you will benefit from *Find Your Focus Zone*.

I *Had* to Study Attention

My career-long interest in attention began in graduate school in the mid-1970s. Completing a doctoral dissertation was not easy for me. While my neighborhood chums were out partying, I had to sit at my desk, read dry professional journals, methodically and meticulously design and conduct research, and produce technical writing. I remember going to see my adviser for his review of the first draft of my master's thesis. "Lucy Jo," he said, "Your writing is so passionate." I beamed, but it was a short-lived moment of glory. "Scientific writing," he continued in a monotone voice, "is *dispassionate*."

To get through this, I needed to figure out how to make myself buckle down and stick with a lot of tedious work. Then it hit me: why not do my dissertation on ways to resist distraction?

At that time, psychologists had just begun to use cognitive methods to help people lift their moods, face fear, decrease anxiety, manage anger, and improve their habits. A cognitive method is a technique to change the way you feel and act by changing the way you think. I wondered if cognitive methods could be used with success to train a person to pay attention. I chose as my topic: "Cognitive Strategies for Self-Control: The Use of Self-Instruction to Resist Distraction."

I put together a tape of highly distracting audio—snippets of juicy gossip, riffs of rock-and-roll, and bits and pieces of stand-up comedy and funny skits. I had to test it first to make sure it was as distracting to others as it was to me. Word got out about my project, and undergraduates lined up outside my office to volunteer for that part of the study!

For the experiment itself, I tested sixty subjects, one by one. I asked each subject to proofread while listening to the distracting tape. I let subjects know they were being observed through a one-way mirror as they read, while they continually underlined text and looked for errors to circle. Behind the mirror, three trained raters with stopwatches measured the amount of time each subject spent at work, and counted the number of "departures from task," that is, the number of times that a subject looked away, paused too long, or lifted his pencil from the page.

Beforehand, each subject had been randomly assigned to one of five groups. I'd trained four of the groups with four different types of cognitive strategies to use while proofreading: (1) A *thought-stopping* self-instruction—silently saying, "No, I will not listen"; or its short form, "No." (2) A *vaccination* model—the same thought-stopping strategy with the same amount of practice time but with the distracting sounds gradually increased from soft to loud during practice. (3) A *goal-visualization* self-instruction—silently saying, "I will do my work"; or its short form, "Work." (4) A *blocking* strategy—humming silently. I didn't train the fifth group; they served as a control.

The subjects in the four groups who received training in any of the cognitive strategies did significantly better than the control subjects with no training. The trained subjects spent more time at work and departed from their tasks fewer times. It didn't seem to matter exactly which cognitive strategy they had been taught. Any strategy worked better than no strategy. I'd probably still be writing the introduction to my dissertation if I had not used cognitive strategies myself.

Your Focus Zone

Since then I've pursued my interest in attention, both in research and practice. I found that most of the progress in improving human attention came from sports psychology, so I decided to advance my knowledge and skills by training with an eight-time Olympic sports psychologist.

I learned that, when it comes to staying focused, elite athletes face two distinct challenges: long, boring hours of practice; and high-stakes, high-pressure events. To map out which cognitive strategies they need for each of these two types of challenges, athletes use an upside-down U curve, which you'll learn about in Chapter 1. At one end of the curve, they're underactivated. In other words, they're not stimulated enough to pay attention, as when they start to train months before a race. Then they need cognitive strategies to psych themselves *up*. At the other end of the curve, athletes are overactivated or too stimulated to concentrate. Typically this happens at the event, as they nervously wait at the starting line. Then they need cognitive strategies to calm themselves *down*. In the middle of the curve, athletes are *in the zone* and have the best control over their attention. Here they use strategies to check on themselves and make sure they stay in a relaxed-alert state.

The upside-down U fits with the results of my doctoral study. All the strategies I taught my subjects worked because they all prevented overstimulation. The subjects' attention improved because they filtered out the interfering sounds of the distracting tape. By limiting their own levels of stimulation, the subjects stayed in their focus zone.

The upside-down U also explains many of the problems people face today when they encounter daily distraction. As our culture has become more mobile, high-speed, techno-stressed, information-cluttered, and media-saturated, we are getting pushed out of our focus zones without even realizing it. We accept as normal a chronic state of being either overactivated or exhausted. We wind up in a continuous state of partial attention in which our choices slip away from us and our quality of life suffers.

For years, I've been helping people of all ages find their focus zones by applying the principles and techniques in this book. I'm pleased and excited now to share these ideas and tools with you, too.

The Age of the Short Attention Span

If I were conducting my doctoral study today, I wonder if I'd even need to play a distracting audiotape. We each have our own internal tapes running on a perpetual loop inside our heads. As you read this, are you also thinking, *Who needs a return call today? . . . Did I check my e-mail? . . . Is my cell phone charged? . . . What time is it? . . . Whose turn is it to cook dinner?* . . . You may even be glancing at your Black-Berry to see if you have a new message. (Do you?)

Digital-age distraction is everywhere. In 1971 the average American was targeted by 560 daily advertising messages. Not counting spam or pop-up ads by 1997, that number increased to more than 3,000 messages per day and it continues to rise. According to a study done at the University of California, Berkeley:

- Worldwide storage of new material has been growing at a rate of over 30 percent a year.
- More than 5 billion instant messages per day were sent in 2002. (AOL began its instant messaging service in 1997.)
- There are 21,264 TV stations in the world, producing 31 million hours of original programming, and 123 million hours of total programming per year.

There has never been a time when taking charge of your attention has been so necessary. Everyone has too much to do and too little time to do it. Downtime has all but disappeared. Someone somewhere is ringing, buzzing, or jabbering from a screen, bringing you dazzling, digitalized distractions to push you further and make you jump faster from . . . what was it you were supposed to be doing? Our need for sleep has gone up, but our time for sleep has gone down. We turn to caffeine and sugar as our stay awake pals, but they sabotage our attention even as they fuel it.

The Benefits of Better Attention

The solutions and strategies in this book will help you to stay on track when the phone rings, the fax hums, and you've got mail. You'll learn skills you can use right away. You'll also be able to teach them to your kids as they cut their teeth on digital distractions.

Imagine feeling confident that coworkers can interrupt, ads pop up on your screen, and impulses jump into your brain, yet you'll stay focused and get your work done on time. Picture the people you care about feeling secure in their knowledge of how much you care, because you listen attentively. Envision taking charge of the way others see you, because you have more awareness of how you look to them.

The skills you learn in *Find Your Focus Zone* will help you:

- Beat procrastination and face boring jobs
- Overcome obstacles and finish what you start
- Prevent yourself from getting overwhelmed and burned out
- Build trust in your close relationships
- Boost your self-confidence
- Increase your efficiency and effectiveness
- Persevere even when you make mistakes

Children Do as We Do (Not as We Say)

I wrote my first book, *Dreamers, Discoverers, and Dynamos* (formerly titled *The Edison Trait*) for parents and teachers. One night, at a workshop, a mother stood up to say, "Dr. Palladino, it's not just kids who are more scatterbrained than ever. It's us, their parents. The adults need help first."

That mom was right on target. In *Find Your Focus Zone*, you'll read about "mirror neurons," one of the most important recent discoveries in brain science. We each have a mirror neuron system that fires identically whether we ourselves perform an action or watch someone else perform it. Mirror neurons might just as well be called "role-model neurons." When your child sees you half-listening, her mirror neuron system fires as if she is half-listening too. When she sees you giving your full attention, her mirror neuron system fires as if she's fully attending as well. In other words, your actions condition hers, automatically and involuntarily.

The great psychologist Carl Jung once said, "If there is anything we wish to change in the child, we should first examine it and see whether it is not something that could better be changed in ourselves." Children's minds are as impressionable as warm wax. If you're a parent, the most compelling reason to improve your own attention might well be to set the best example possible for your child.

In the Chapters Ahead

Find Your Focus Zone is divided into four parts. In Part I, you'll learn about your focus zone, the upside-down U curve, and the link between learning and brain pathways to pay attention. Part II covers emotional, mental, and behavior skills and gives you eight sets of keys, so you can choose the strategies that will work best for you.

⚙ The Eight Keychains

Keychain 1 ⚙ Self-Awareness

Keychain 2 ⚙ Change of State

Keychain 3 ⚙ Procrastination Busters

Keychain 4 ⚙ Anti-Anxiety

Keychain 5 ⚙ Intensity Control

Keychain 6 ⚙ Motivate Yourself

Keychain 7 ⚙ Stay on Track

Keychain 8 ⚙ Healthy Habits

Part III teaches you how to use these keys to unlock success in our digital age of distraction—how to handle interruption and overload in the workplace, how to work from home or in transit, and what to do if you or someone you care about has attention deficit disorder (ADD). In Part IV, you'll learn how to teach your kids to pay attention and what it takes to stay successful as attention becomes even scarcer in our world today.

The Appendix gives you a quick guide to the eight keychains, and lists the three keys on each keychain. In the Resources section, you'll find books, articles, and websites, including sources for the main studies that are described in the book. Additional resources are available at www.yourfocuszone.com.

To be gender friendly, I've used male and female pronouns in alternating chapters throughout the book. I distributed these pronouns evenly when referring to children in Chapter 13—a chapter of particular interest to parents and teachers.

The stories from Chapter 2 of Joe, Meg, and Todd include elements of several people's stories from my practice. The other stories in the book are true, but with fictional names and identifying information.

Attention Is How We Create

Attention is power. If you ever want to see that power in action, try paying attention to a child while her sister or brother is in the same room! In today's world, as the amount and availability of information explode, the value of attention skyrockets. In describing the new "attention economy," business experts Thomas Davenport and John Beck observe, "Companies that succeed in the future will be those expert not in time management, but in attention management."

Attention is the singular act of creativity that is available to each of us every waking moment. We can use it at any time to reward our own behavior and the behavior of others. Behavior that is rewarded will be repeated. Parents and teachers see dramatic differences when they stop giving children attention for disruptive behavior and start catching them at being good. Spouses influence each other's behaviors by what they pay attention to and what they ignore.

Learning to direct your attention empowers you. The more you control the demands on your attention, the less those demands control you. You exert authority over the court of your life and decide what you let in and what you keep out. The Spanish philosopher José Ortega y Gasset once said, "Tell me to what you pay attention and I will tell you who you are."

We create ourselves by what we choose to notice. Whatever we put our attention on develops and grows. A Cherokee elder was teaching the children of the tribe. He told them, "A fight is going on inside of me. It is a terrible battle, and it is between two wolves. One wolf represents fear, anger, guilt, greed, and senselessness. The other stands for faith, peace, truth, love, and reason. The same fight is going on inside you, and inside every other person too." The children thought about it for a while and one child asked the wise man, "Which wolf will win?" The old Cherokee replied, "The one you feed."

Part I

Understanding
Your Focus Zone

In these chapters, you'll learn about your focus zone and the type of strategies you need to pay attention in today's world of distraction. You'll read stories about people from my practice with problems that have kept them outside their focus zones. Part I teaches you about the upside-down U curve and the importance of regulating your own stimulation and drive. You'll also learn about "use it or lose it" brain pathways and see why it's vital to strengthen your neural connections to select and sustain attention.

1

What Is Your Focus Zone?

*Any man who can drive safely while kissing a pretty girl is
simply not giving the kiss the attention it deserves.*

—ALBERT EINSTEIN

In 1977, I was thrown from a horse when it bolted. I suffered a head concussion, had seven stitches across my scalp, and had to wear a cast on my leg for eight weeks. I lost my interest in horseback riding. Twenty-seven years later, my daughter told me she wanted to ride a horse. She was just a few years younger than I was when I had my accident. It seemed the time had come for me to get back on a horse. I found a dude ranch in Santa Barbara where we could ride scenic trails together all day with a small group and a guide.

The morning of the ride we assembled at the stables. To choose the right horse for each of us, the wrangler asked for our experience level. My face must have betrayed my fear. Both my daughter and I had replied, "Beginner," but he gave Rocket to her, and I got Nellie. Momentarily, I felt relieved.

As I mounted, I looked down, and the distance to the ground made me dizzy. My heart pounded and my hands sweat. From his horse, the guide began to instruct us. I was aware he was talking; I knew his words were important. But to my ears, he could have been speaking in Wookie. My focus was scattered like dew on grass. My muscles tensed. My thoughts swirled. Deep inside, a part of me cried, "Get down now while you have the chance!" An opposite part

15

of me planted my feet in my stirrups. Mentally paralyzed, I sat there staring, like a deer in headlights. The guide turned his horse to face the trail and led the other riders as they clip-clopped away, single file. I followed in a fog, with no clue what to do.

After a few minutes on the trail, I calmed myself down. I felt safe again and regained my focus. I trotted up next to my daughter, who recapped for me what the guide had said. The day turned out beautifully. But thinking back to the corral, when everything had been a blur, I wondered, how could I have lost my attention at the moment I needed it most? And how did I get it back?

A Critical Connection

The link between *attention and stimulation* is well established. This relationship is the core of understanding attention and learning how to control it. Attention is poor when you are either understimulated or overstimulated. Attention is best when your level of stimulation is just right.

Psychologists use the term "arousal level" to describe how bored or excited you feel. It is a physiological term that corresponds to how much or how little adrenaline is pumping through your system. The amount of adrenaline, in turn, depends on how bored or excited you feel. Arousal is also called activation or drive.

Arousal and adrenaline create a chicken-and-egg cycle: the more excited you feel, the more adrenaline you pump; the more adrenaline you pump, the more excited you feel. The boring side of the story works the same way. The less excited you feel, the less adrenaline you pump; and the less adrenaline you pump, the less excited you feel. Either way—over- or underactivated—your attention suffers.

When you're *over*stimulated and your adrenaline level is too high, you're in overdrive. Depending on your thoughts and situation, you might feel intense, overexcited, worried, nervous, angry, or afraid. Think of the first few moments when you have to give a speech, take a test, or face a confrontation. Your heart beats harder, your breathing gets shallow, and you feel like your brain has left the building.

When you're *under*stimulated and your adrenaline level is too low, you're underpowered; you lack sufficient drive. You might feel stuck, slow, or unmotivated. Picture having to write a technical report, clean a cluttered closet, or do your taxes. It's hard to keep your mind on what you're doing. You feel sluggish and sleepy, with a strong urge to check your e-mail, watch TV, or grab a snack—anything to avoid the boring task at hand.

When stimulation is just right, you're in a relaxed-alert state: your muscles are relaxed and your mind is alert. Attention experts call this relaxed-alert state "optimal arousal"—you have an ideal level of drive. You have adequate stimulation and the right amount of adrenaline, and you feel motivated, confident, and focused. Envision doing something you genuinely like to do—reading a novel that is a page-turner, going on a nature walk, or traveling to some interesting new place. You have a sense of clarity and involvement. Paying attention in a relaxed-alert state is practically effortless.

Let's return to the day I was horseback riding. Imagine that one of the other riders was so experienced that the guide's instructions added no new information. That rider would be bored—underdriven—and would have a tough time concentrating on what the

	DRIVE LEVEL		
	Underpowered	**Overdrive**	**Optimal**
Stimulation	too low	too high	adequate
Adrenaline	too low	too high	balanced
State	bored	overexcited	relaxed-alert
Feelings	apathy	anxiety	confidence
	fatigue	fear	interest
	passivity	pressure	activity
	spaciness	stress	clarity
	indecision	irritability	motivation
Attention	poor	poor	best

guide was saying. In contrast, I was at the other end of the spectrum entirely. I was in overdrive. My brain was a firestorm of adrenaline, and my concentration was shot. At either extreme, under- or over-driven, your best attention is out of reach.

When the level of your drive is just right, you feel sharp and able to concentrate. The other riders, like my daughter, focused easily on the guide. They were excited by the ride, but not frightened or immobilized. They were stirred to listen, but not in a swirl, as I was. In their relaxed-alert state, they could pay full attention to the guide, their horses, and the breathtaking beauty of a coastline trail overlooking the Pacific Ocean. Good attention has its rewards!

The Upside-Down U Curve

To understand the relationship between attention and stimulation, picture a simple graph that looks like a hill or an upside-down U. Attention is the vertical axis, increasing upward from worst to best. Stimulation is the horizontal axis, increasing left to right, from low to high.

The left end (going uphill) represents understimulation, and the right end (going downhill) stands for overstimulation. At both ends, under- and overstimulation, your attention is at its worst. In the center (the middle of the hill), stimulation is just right and your attention is at its best. *This is your focus zone.*

It feels good to be in your zone, where stimulation is sufficient and steady. In this relaxed-alert state of body and mind, you feel effective and get things done with a power that lasts. You listen well, sustain attention, organize efficiently, make sound decisions, and finish what you start.

The inverted U has been in the psychological literature for about a century. It illustrates the Yerkes-Dodson law developed by Robert M. Yerkes, PhD and John D. Dodson, PhD in 1908 to explain the results of a series of experiments. The law states that performance (or attention) increases with arousal (or stimulation) but only up to a certain point. When arousal level gets too high, performance decreases.

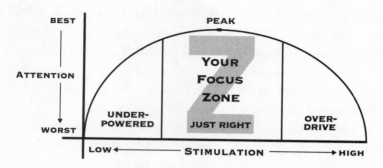

Your Focus Zone on the Upside-Down U Curve

Through the years, the upside-down U has continued to serve as a unifying principle to explain findings in biopsychology and neuroscience. Research studies have confirmed and expanded this classic curvilinear relationship to include more complex variations. It's a core teaching in sports psychology, and it is used by world-class athletes as a model to practice attention control.

Sometimes the horizontal axis—stimulation—is labeled drive, intensity, motivation, level of adrenaline, or physiological arousal. And sometimes the vertical axis—attention—is labeled selective attention, concentration, focus, mental performance, or performance efficiency. The center range—your focus zone—has also been called the optimal range of performance, the individual zone of optimal functioning (IZOF), and, in sports, the zone.

At the very top of the hill, the exact center resembles a peak. The closer you get to this peak, the closer you get to an ideal state of stimulation and attention. Athletes have long referred to this state as "peak performance." Experts in creativity call it "flow," and describe it as an altered state of consciousness. The term was coined by Mihaly Csikszentmihalyi, PhD, who collected data on thousands of highly focused individuals, mountain climbers to chess players. The word "flow" best described their experience when they engaged in self-controlled, goal-related, meaningful actions. Csikszentmihalyi explained it further as a suspension of time and the freedom to get totally absorbed in what you're doing. Artists, musicians, and inventors strive to achieve flow, the pinnacle of the relaxed-alert state.

Although reaching this peak state is ideal for single-purpose undivided attention, it can be tough to achieve and impractical in the workplace, which is both clock- and interruption-driven. Fortunately, you don't have to reach this peak to be in your focus zone. When you're anywhere in the center range on the graph, your attention is engaged and you are productive.

Being in your focus zone is a matter of degree. Sometimes you'll be closer to peak performance (in the center) and sometimes you'll be closer to feeling under- or overstimulated (at each end).

Being under- or overstimulated is also a matter of degree. You could be a little bored or intolerably bored, or a little hyper or very hyper. But if you're anywhere outside your zone, you're likely to run into trouble. Have you ever been at a meeting or lecture when your thoughts start to wander? You may not have spaced out completely, but you missed some of the details. Now you're stuck with the problem of worrying if they were important to you or not.

Mild forms of overstimulation cause problems too. Have you ever felt anxious while taking an exam? You probably got a lower grade because your concentration was weakened. You didn't flunk, but you felt frustrated, since you knew you'd studied hard and had the answers somewhere in your mind. They would have come to you more easily if you'd been in your focus zone.

Being in Your Zone

When it comes to paying attention, your zone is definitely the place to be. We've all been there at some time, and when we are, it feels great. Think of the last time you were doing something you genuinely like to do—a pet project, hobby, or sport. You might have been researching a favorite topic, organizing your music, or conversing with a friend. Remember what it felt like to be engaged in what you were doing—relaxed, yet energized? You may recall feeling a pleasant sense of purpose, meaning, and motivation. You may even have thought to yourself, "I wish it could be like this all the time."

The good news is that most of the time it can be. With practice, you can teach yourself how to stay in your zone. Like Olympic athletes who practice psychological skills, *you can stay in your focus zone by choice.* This is true whether you're working on some truly boring task or at the other extreme, facing a once-in-a-lifetime moment of high-stakes tension. Top performers have trained themselves to do this reliably and you can, too.

Understanding Overstimulation

First, let's take a closer look at what happens when you're overexcited. When most people think of an adrenaline rush, they imagine euphoria, like the thrill of a roller-coaster ride. We pay money to ride on a roller coaster. It's fun. We regard this experience as desirable.

But "overstimulation" refers to the total state of your brain and body when you're pumping too much adrenaline, and usually that's undesirable. Your heart beats faster and your focus either bounces around or gets stuck in one place. A roller-coaster ride is an exception. You can scream and still smile because the rational part of your brain knows you're safe and not actually on a train going over a cliff.

Usually, in an overstimulated state, fear is *not* your friend. Your perception of fear triggers a fight-or-flight response in the survival part of your brain, whether this response is helpful to you or not. Even knowing the fun that lies ahead, have you ever felt the sudden urge to duck out the exit gate when it's your turn to step onto the roller coaster? That's adrenaline fueling your impulse to flee.

In other fear-evoking situations, the survival part of your brain pumps adrenaline because it assumes you'll need to fight. You may be preparing to have a difficult meeting with your boss, and you sense that you may lose status or money. The survival part of your brain reacts to this danger as though you have to fight off an attack from a wild animal. It pumps adrenaline to increase your physical strength and give hair-trigger speed to your reflexes.

Signs of mild fight or flight in your thoughts, words, or actions are flags that you're going into overdrive. Common signs of fight include feeling cranky, argumentative, or overly critical of yourself or others. Common signs of flight include worry, anxiety, and rumination, although the connection between these feelings and the impulse to flee may not be as readily apparent. These feelings result when the survival part of your brain wants you to get away, but you're at work or caught in traffic and you can't get up and leave. Without realizing it, you do the only thing a trapped person can do—you escape in your mind. You flee mentally from the reality of the here and now, with adrenaline-fueled thoughts of past, future, or even imagined fears and mistakes.

Different Activities, Different Zones

Every activity has its own zone or optimal state of adrenaline-fueled drive. At game time, an NFL linebacker needs to pump a lot more adrenaline than you do when you sit down to write your quarterly sales report. Generally speaking, physical activities require more adrenaline, which sends strength to the body to physically fight or flee. Mental activities require less adrenaline because adrenaline gives the body extra physical strength by diverting blood flow away from the brain. For mental activities, the brain wants all the blood flow it can get.

In sports psychology, the zone for each sport is determined by its ratio of physical strength to mental skill. Boxing, for example, requires force and might, so the optimal adrenaline level for boxing is high. Tennis or golf demands great concentration, so the optimal adrenaline level is much lower. In the language of sports psychology, the inverted U curve for boxing is higher on the arousal continuum than it is for tennis or golf. Being in the zone is important for all athletes, but the levels that define the zone itself depend on the demands of the particular sport.

In your own life, the levels that define your zone depend on what you're doing and how much—or how little—adrenaline it demands. Nearly all information-age jobs require mostly mental activity. Gathering data, managing spreadsheets, writing reports, teleconferencing, and creating computer code are mental, not physical, tasks. When you sit at your desk or your computer to concentrate, you perform better with less adrenaline. A construction worker who is lifting, digging, and hammering all day needs more.

During the course of a day as you go from activity to activity, the amount of adrenaline you need to stay in your focus zone changes. If you're conducting a sales conference, you need animation and passion more than attention to detail. If you're reviewing the wording of a contract, it's just the opposite. Sometimes, you need to shift quickly. If you're giving a presentation, you want fire in your voice; but then during the question-and-answer period, it's time for careful listening, accurate recall, and concise responses.

Have you ever been in a conversation when someone said something a bit intrusive or asked you a pointed question, and you felt mildly threatened or provoked? You couldn't come up with an incisive answer and may even have felt brain locked. That's because an immediate shot of adrenaline had kicked you into a hyperalert state. Later on—usually in the shower—you thought of exactly what you wished you had said at that moment. This is because you returned to a relaxed-alert state. You came back to your focus zone.

A Two-Step Process

When you're not in your zone and you lose control of your attention, what's actually happening is that your adrenaline level is wrong for your current situation. Your brain is pumping either too much or too little adrenaline to get the job done.

Fortunately, you have choices. Like an elite athlete, *you can reclaim your attention by getting back into your focus zone*. You can use your thoughts, feelings, and actions to change your adrenaline level.

Remember the chicken-and-egg cycle: too much stimulation causing too much adrenaline, and so on? Well, the good news is that you *can* break this cycle. Using the same psychological skills that elite athletes use, you can increase or decrease your stimulation as needed, and adjust the adrenaline levels inside your brain. You can return to a relaxed-alert state and get back in charge of your own attention.

Think of any sport that requires balance—skating, skiing, bicycling. At speeds that are either too slow or fast, you do not feel in control no matter how hard you try. Regaining control becomes a two-step process. First you need to realize that you're losing control. Then you need to speed up or slow down to regain your balance.

When you feel distracted, bored, or provoked, regaining your attention is also a two-step process. First you need to realize that you're out of your zone. Then you need to apply a skill or a strategy to get back in. There are many ways to do this. In Part II, you'll learn key methods for the situations you face every day.

TO REGAIN LOST ATTENTION

Step 1. Stop and notice you're no longer in your focus zone.

Step 2. Choose a strategy to either rev up or calm down.

The eight keychains give you effective ways to do both.

Is Multitasking Good or Bad?

In today's world, we all multitask. As you read this, are you also munching on a snack, listening to music, or maybe flying to Chicago? The burning question of our time is: does all this multitasking help or hurt?

The upside-down U addresses this question. If you're underpowered, multitasking is good because an additional activity adds stimulation and gets you into your focus zone. Let's say you're crunching some code and your mind starts to wander. You notice you're getting bored, so you open a window on the bottom of your screen and download some rock music videos to glance at and keep you pumped as you work. The added stim(ulation) gets you back into your zone.

At the other end of the curve, if you're in overdrive, multitasking will only make matters worse. Let's say you're working on a project under deadline. Other members of the team constantly call, text, e-mail, instant-message, and even walk up to your desk to interrupt you. Your mind is racing, and you may feel the impulse to download some rock videos, but the added stim will cost you in performance and productivity.

It can also happen that you're crunching code, you get bored, and you download a rock video that's so awesome you can't stop watching it. You've increased your stimulation but you've added too much. By overshooting your focus zone, you trade one problem for another. Now you're caught in a time-wasting cycle of attention swings from one end of the upside-down U to the other.

The video ends and you're overexcited, but it's time to get back to work. You try, but compared to the rock video, the code is even more boring than before. You make yourself work on it but soon you start to chat or check e-mail in another window. Again, multitasking gives you a spurt of stimulation. But again, you're too pumped to crunch code. You get absorbed in checking out the jokes and links your buddies sent you, until you notice the clock. You try one more time to force yourself to face the code, which, in contrast, is now more boring than ever. You hang in there as long as you can, then give up and check your RSS feed to post comments on your favorite blogs. What you could have done in an hour has taken half a day.

Mindful Multitasking

The key to multitasking is to use it strategically. This can be a challenge, because it's hard to be honest with ourselves when it comes to stimulation. As you'll learn in Chapter 3, our brains are biased toward stimulants whether they're good for us or not.

Take cell phones, for example. About 75 percent of all drivers report using their phone while driving. We like to talk and drive. Yet research using driving simulators reveals that when drivers are on cell phones, they're more likely to be in traffic accidents, miss more traffic signals, and react more slowly. We ignore what researchers call "inattention blindness"—missing important cues when our attention is incomplete. The stim centers in our brains prefer that we don't know we're at risk, because we're drawn to the stim of driving and talking.

Does this mean you should never use your cell phone when driving? In today's world, how impractical is that? A commonsense approach is to keep the upside-down U in mind. Use a hands-free set and be aware of the impact of adding more stimulation to each situation that you're in. Ask yourself what it's doing to your ability to stay in your focus zone.

Mindful multitasking is one of the keys on the change-of-state keychain that you'll learn about in Chapter 5. Mindful multitasking means that you consciously check in with yourself and determine the focus zone you need for each new situation—in your car; at your desk; or with your family, friends, or coworkers. Every situation requires its own judgment call. Sometimes you'll choose to multitask and sometimes you won't. But with mindful multitasking, you don't automatically answer a ring, beep, or interrupting voice. You make a deliberate decision based on reason and strategy.

Psych Up or Settle Down?

Finding your focus zone isn't always easy. Not only does it change from activity to activity, but it's different from one person to the next. Personality, physiology, style of thinking, age, and experience are all factors. You may not be able to talk, e-mail, and instant-message at the same time, but your child probably can. And in your child's classroom, while some students get distracted by papers rattling, chairs moving, and classmates whispering, others do not.

Just as we each have a different face and different fingerprints, we each have a different brain chemistry. Your adrenaline thresholds are unique to you. The way in which *you* metabolize adrenaline determines your relationship with stimulation, and your own, personal focus zone.

As you read *Find Your Focus Zone*, you'll get better at recognizing when you're in your zone or not, and what to do to stay there. Sometimes, you may feel as if you're underpowered, but the deeper problem is *too much* adrenaline. Procrastination is a good example.

Let's say you're postponing straightening out your finances, or getting the information you need to make a health-related decision.

On the surface it looks like you just don't want to sit down and start a low-stim job like organizing or doing research. But deep down you're scared. You're afraid of how much debt you might be in, or of possibly needing a risky operation. Fear and the adrenaline that goes with it stop you before you even get the chance to face boredom as a problem. Before you can go forward, you need to deal with your fear calmly and get back into your focus zone.

Many capable parents have come to my office bewildered by what happens at homework time. The harder they try to get their child to sit down and focus, the more the child argues, gets upset, or spaces out. Trying to act responsibly, they'll threaten to ground their child or take privileges away. But this does not get the child fired up to work. Instead the child gets immobilized or has a meltdown.

The problem is that the child's arguing, upset, and spaciness are signs of a fight-or-flight response—a result of his unacknowledged fear. On the outside, the child might look bored or defiant. But on the inside, even though he himself may not realize it, he's scared he can't do it, will make mistakes, or won't do as well as his peers. He's got too much, not too little adrenaline pumping. His parents' threat just makes him pump even more and pushes him farther out of his focus zone. Instead of getting motivated, the child gets overwhelmed.

Back at the ranch, scared stiff in the saddle, I may have looked like my mind was a million miles away and I was bored. But if someone had yelled at me to pay attention, I probably would've burst into tears. I needed to lower my adrenaline level so I could regain concentration. I had to keep my panic in check—and ride it out— until I relaxed enough to get back into my focus zone.

Bored, Hyper, or Both

*When a player comes to recognize that learning to focus
may be more valuable to him than a backhand, he shifts
from being primarily a player of the outer game to being
a player of the Inner Game. Then, instead of learning
to focus to improve his tennis, he practices tennis
to improve his focus.*

—W. TIMOTHY GALLWEY

A perennial favorite, *The Inner Game of Tennis* teaches the secret of staying focused on the court: let go of pressure and relax. Gallwey names the voice of self-criticism as the number-one enemy of focused play: "I should have gotten that one," "I should be quicker on my feet," "I should take my racket back lower in my backswing." These "shoulds" knock you out of your focus zone into both ends of the upside-down U curve. At one extreme, they cause tension, so you feel worried and anxious. At the other, they rob you of the joy of play, so you also feel bored and underpowered.

In today's world, we have our own set of shoulds: "I should work faster and get more done," "I should make more money than I'm making," "I should have closed that deal, made that call, sold that stock." As in tennis, these "shoulds" create both tension and boredom. They swing you back and forth from over- to understimulated.

The swings start when you drive yourself too hard, and then you burn out, feel unmotivated, and lose your focus. Feeling low, you blame yourself. Then, to stop feeling guilty, you drive yourself even harder. Riding an attention swing like this, you feel like a yo-yo. You pass through your focus zone, but you don't get to stay there very long.

Attention swings are symptomatic of digital-age distraction, but everyone has a different style. While most people swing back and forth, some lean more toward one side of the upside-down U or the other. Remember the three lists of questions in the Introduction? Did you find that one described you better than the others—having attention swings, being scattered and spacey, or being hyperfast and hyperfocused?

In this chapter, you'll read about Joe, Meg, and Todd, whose stories are based on people I've seen in my practice. Joe has attention swings. Meg is too scattered and spacey. And Todd is too hyperfast and hyperfocused.

You'll relate to some but not all aspects of these profiles. And you'll see glimpses of people you know, but with differences, too. Even though we're each individual, we're alike enough to learn from one another.

Attention Swings Miss the Zone

Joe is a brilliant engineer at a small high-tech company. He has a reputation as the man to see if you've got a tough problem to solve, but only if you catch him at the right time. Joe has trouble getting started. In the morning, he just can't settle down and concentrate. Lost in thought, Joe wanders to the coffee machine, then sits down and surfs the net until he's focused enough to work. Not long after he gets back from lunch, Joe is in the same half-present state.

On the other hand, if there's a crisis or an exciting new project, Joe comes alive. When a virus caused the servers to crash, Joe stayed up all night and got the network back online. But after that, Joe got fascinated with virus code and continued to analyze it at the expense of his ongoing projects.

At meetings, Joe gets restless and can't resist text messaging and checking e-mail. He gets involved with his messages and misses the discussion. His ideas have greatly helped his company, yet Joe gets mixed performance reviews instead of the outstanding ones that his contributions deserve.

At home, it seems Joe has just the opposite problem. He'd rather start something new than finish what he's begun. His computer desk is stacked with papers and discs, he's still wiring his home entertainment system, and he's promised prints of photos to family members and friends from several Christmases ago. Joe likes to surf the net and play video games. He gets so engrossed that if his wife calls him for dinner or his kids ask for help with their homework, he snaps at them. That's why he does it late at night, after everyone else is in bed.

Joe says he can't clear his computer desk until he has a long enough block of time to do it; he wants more information before he makes final decisions on the home entertainment system; and he can't print photos until he's cleared his computer desk. On a typical Saturday morning, Joe looks at all he has to do, feels overwhelmed, and doesn't make much headway on his ongoing projects. What he'd really like to do is get some new multimedia software so he can make cool home videos, but he's afraid to tell his wife.

Under- *and* Overstimulated

Joe is a poster boy for digital-age distraction. He spends the first few hours of each workday on the understimulated side of the upside-down U curve. He is too bored to do his job. When he faces the novelty of a new project or a threat like a computer virus, his adrenaline surges and kicks him into his focus zone. Joe doesn't stay there long, though. He goes into an overstimulated state and can't shift his focus back to his usual job.

At meetings, Joe gets caught in the same kind of pendulum swing. He gets bored with the discussion, then overstimulated checking messages, then even more bored trying to get back into a discussion that no longer involves him.

At home, when Joe is bored, he starts a new project. The adrenaline he gets from the novelty of it keeps him in his zone for a while, but soon he's bored again. He bounces from one unfinished project to the next, without the benefit of feeling the satisfaction that comes from completing a job. Because he's not in his focus zone, Joe stalls on making decisions, and self-doubt gets the better of him. He longs to escape his boredom and indecision by doing what he does best: start a new project.

The habit of staying up late at night is a big contributor to Joe's attention swings. Joe is conditioned to his late-night stim and he likes it. He feels alive and free, with no one telling him what to do. But lack of sleep causes Joe to greet each new day on the understimulated side of the curve. To get himself going, Joe drinks coffee and eats doughnuts. This propels him into an overstimulated state. Joe gets his work done, but not without cost. As the effects of the caffeine and sugar wear off, he nosedives into an understimulated state after lunch. Joe continues to swing back and forth all day, using coffee and sweets as stimulants that kick him from one side of the upside-down U to the other.

Overstimulation Can Make You Too Hyper*fast*

Overstimulation looks different at different times, and Joe is a good example. At home on Saturday morning, when Joe feels overstimulated, his mind races and he gets too hyperfast. His adrenaline gives him a big boost of energy, but he squanders it jumping from one project to the next. If you talk with Joe when he's in this state, he'll tell you his future plans to expand his projects. While his propensity for brainstorming is a valuable asset, Joe gets stuck in his idea-generating mode when it's time to settle down to business.

I've chosen the words "too hyperfast" to communicate that, in the big picture, this extreme is ineffective and inefficient. Although being hyperfast sounds like a very good thing—a kind of superpower you wish for when there's work to be done—being too hyperfast is wasteful and unsustainable. You lose your ability to stay focused to the finish. And even if you force yourself to stick with one project, you quickly burn out and fall into an attention swing.

Overstimulation Can Make You Too Hyper*focused*

Late at night, when Joe is overstimulated, or when he starts a new project at work, Joe gets hyper in a different way—he gets into an intense state of being too hyperfocused. His high level of adrenaline *narrows* his attention. He gets glued to what he is doing, unable to see the bigger picture. Surfing the net or watching video games, Joe forgets the time, his need for sleep, and his commitment to his family. At work, when he starts a new project, he neglects his routine responsibilities.

Again, I use the term "too hyperfocused" because being hyperfocused is a useful skill and a desirable state. But an overstimulated state of being too hyperfocused is more like getting super glued stuck. You can't move on without ungluing yourself first. In this restrictive state of overstimulation, Joe can't stop focusing on one and only one thing, and is headed for burnout and attention swings.

Being Too Hyperfocused Is *Not* Flow or Peak Performance

When Joe is engrossed surfing the net or playing video games, to an outside observer he looks as if he's in his focus zone. He's so absorbed in what he's doing that he appears to be in a state of flow, the type of peak performance identified by Mihaly Csikszentmihalyi described in Chapter 1.

In a number of ways, being too hyperfocused looks like flow: total concentration, deep involvement, a sense of challenge, and losing track of time. But the critical difference is the *presence of tension* in a state of extreme hyperfocus. In contrast, when you're in a state of flow or peak performance, you remain relaxed.

In extreme hyperfocus, adrenaline builds. Your intensity locks you into a narrow field of focus and takes away your freedom of choice. You keep a white-knuckled grip on what you're doing, and start to devalue other activities, even ones you usually like. The stirrings of addiction are not far from the surface.

On the other hand, flow or peak performance is the pinnacle of your focus zone, a *relaxed*-alert state. Attention flows easily because just the right amount of adrenaline is pumping. Csikszentmihalyi describes it as a calm state of balance and joy, characterized by openness, flexibility, and freedom of thought.

Too Hyperfocused vs. Flow

	Too Hyperfocused	Flow
State	tense	relaxed
Accepts Mistakes	no	yes
Sustainable	no	yes

So when Joe is at his computer at night, how can he tell if he's trapped in an overaroused state of hyperfocus or enjoying a relaxed state of flow? One way is his reaction to frustration. If he finds himself able to accept mistakes and setbacks, he's probably in a state of flow. But if he slams his joystick because the action just got frantic in his video game, he's overstimulated and too hyperfocused.

Another tip-off is how well Joe allows for reasonable interruption. When you're in your zone, you certainly don't want to be interrupted, but if you are and the interruption is for a good cause, you can accept it in an amicable way. Without meaning to, Joe scowls at his family so that they'll leave him alone. This is a sign that he's pumping too much adrenaline and is too hyperfocused. If, on the other hand, Joe could leave his games with a good attitude, it would be a sign that he had been in his focus zone.

Scattered and Spacey Miss the Zone

Meg is a graphic artist in business for herself. She has a reputation for her ability to use color and design in unique ways. But Meg has difficulty with administrative details and finishing work on time. Although she makes a decent income, she spends it on late fees and penalties for missed deadlines. Sometimes she loses customers who like her and her work, but need their jobs done faster than she can deliver.

Most of the other graphic artists use their computers to keep track of their business. They've streamlined bookkeeping tasks like printing invoices and paying bills. Meg knows she needs to start using an electronic spreadsheet, but just hasn't gotten around to it yet.

Meg lives in an apartment downtown. She seldom has guests because her place is a mess. As an artist, she feels frustrated, because this offends her aesthetic sensibilities. Nonetheless, she lives with rooms full of clutter and stacks of sketchbooks and magazines everywhere. Her closets and drawers are a conglomeration of whatever was lying around the last time she cleaned.

Meg has many friends and she enjoys doing them favors. It seems that every time she blocks out time to reorganize her home, friends call to ask her to help redecorate theirs. Meg readily agrees because she likes to feel needed and figures she can always clean her own apartment some other time.

Like Joe and all the rest of us in the digital age of distraction, Meg has attention swings. Sometimes when she's creating new designs, she isolates herself for days and doesn't answer her door, phone, or e-mail. Then, when she finishes, she goes out with friends, or stays in and visits chat rooms until dawn the next morning. But although Meg has some attention swings, most of the time she's at the underpowered end of the upside-down U.

After the creative phase of a project is done, Meg has a hard time with low stim jobs such as measuring, figuring out dimensions, and writing detailed instructions for the printer. She runs low on adrenaline and puts off boring tasks like writing up her orders and invoices. These chores pile up and hang over her head like a dark shadow. Although she's bright and resourceful, Meg hasn't yet computerized her tasks, because she seldom has time to do anything but catch up. Knowing she's constantly behind, having to apologize and pay late fees, Meg feels a little guilty almost all the time.

Doing favors for her friends gives Meg an instant reprieve from her guilt over her procrastination. While she's helping others, Meg's adrenaline levels perk up and she regains her focus. That's why, when friends call, she says yes the way a thirsty person drinks water.

Meg goes out with friends often—to movies, restaurants, and the theater. She enjoys the release this gives her. But when Meg comes home, her adrenaline goes down again, and her focus gets as muddled as her closets and drawers.

Too Hyperfast and Too Hyperfocused Miss the Zone

Todd is a finance officer who is young for his high-level position. Ambitious and hardworking, he rose rapidly in his field. Although some might call him a type A workaholic, Todd protests. "You don't know what a type A workaholic is unless you've met my dad." Todd's dad spent most of his time at the office. Except for major holidays, he missed family meals.

Because Todd didn't get to know his own dad, he promised himself he would not be an absent dad, too. And in his mind, he's not. Although he's responsible for managing millions of dollars in assets, Todd still makes it a priority to spend time with his family.

Todd lives in California, but does business on a daily basis with people in New York. Because of the time difference, he starts his day early. Every morning, Todd brings his laptop to the breakfast table, and tracks stock quotes and instant messages while the family eats together. He prides himself in his ability to do his work and still be with his children, unlike his own father. Todd rapidly shifts his focus from computer screen to kitchen table, although sometimes a stock ticker or sudden price change grabs his attention and he gets totally absorbed in his work.

At the office, when an employee he supervises comes in to talk, Todd keeps one eye on his monitor, on the lookout for incoming messages. When a big deal is coming through, everyone knows enough to stay out of Todd's way.

At school, Todd's older daughter, Becky, has poor concentration. Her teacher thinks she may have attention deficit disorder. When the school counselor asks her why she doesn't listen in the classroom, she argues and insists that she does. Becky says she is multitasking like her dad and that it's a waste of time to sit in the classroom and not be getting something else done too. Recently,

Becky wasn't invited on a sleepover with the other girls in her class. Todd's wife has seen her acting bossy with other children. The school counselor suspects low self-esteem.

Todd has a high tolerance for adrenaline. So did his dad and so does his daughter. Todd gets a lot done; he is a skillful multitasker. But once Todd gets his motor started, he drives himself right past his focus zone, directly into an overstimulated state. His focus gets narrowed and Todd, his coworkers, and his family pay the price.

When it comes to his family, Todd's intentions are good as gold. But this does not mean that the results of his actions are what he intends them to be. When Todd multitasks at the breakfast table, his daughter's mirror neurons—the brain mechanism for learning from a model—are firing away. Automatically and with no one realizing it, Todd's daughter is learning to mirror the pattern of her dad's divided attention.

Something else is happening at the breakfast table, too. Every so often Todd gives his laptop his full attention when an urgent matter comes up. From his daughter's point of view, Dad's attention can be lost suddenly and unpredictably at any moment. Most kids are resilient and tough-skinned enough to accept a normal amount of rejection from other kids on the playground. But no child is built to handle a parent's rejection at home. Nature designs children to care deeply about their father's attentiveness to them. A child who at any moment might feel ignored by the most important man in her life has to build stronger-than-average defenses. Becky's budding self-esteem takes a hit with each flash of unintentional rejection from her dad.

Except for a mild sense of ennui, Todd feels very little motivation to change. He's making a ton of money and he's always got a deal going on. The employees he supervises at work dislike having to walk on eggshells with him, but they know better than to tell him so. His daughter may act up, but Todd doesn't see any connection between her behavior problems and him. Being such a high achiever himself, Todd doesn't really believe his daughter has low self-esteem.

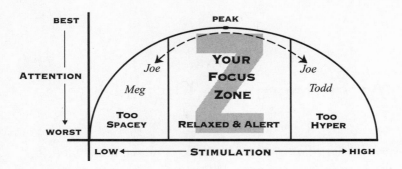

Picturing Joe, Meg, and Todd on the Upside-Down U Curve.
Where Do You Place Yourself?

Bored, Hyper, or in the Zone?

Do you have attention swings like Joe? Do you feel scattered and spacey like Meg? Or do you get too hyperfast and too hyperfocused like Todd? In our distraction-saturated culture, there's some combination of Joe, Meg, and Todd in every one of us. We spend a lot of time missing the zone.

Why is this so? What's happening to our attention today? Chapter 3 looks at why we have attention swings and get stuck at the extremes of the upside-down U curve.

3

Attention in the Digital Age

A weekday edition of the New York Times *contains more information than the average person was likely to come across in a lifetime in 17th century England.*

—RICHARD SAUL WURMAN

Electronic stimulation is changing the way we pay attention. To understand what it's doing to us and to our children, let's look at what we know about human attention.

There are two main kinds of attention: selective and sustained. Selective attention is sometimes called filtering. Sustained attention is also called concentration or attention span.

Selective Attention

We are constantly bombarded with sights, sounds, and smells from the outside world, as well as thoughts, impulses, and emotions from inside our brains and bodies. Stop reading for a moment. Look up and consider all the stimuli coming at you right now—the lights and colors around you, ambient noise, nagging thoughts of things you have to do, emotional memories of recent events. Do you need to swallow? Scratch an itch? Shift your weight in the chair? It is a feat of nature that you can block all this out and return to the printed words on this page. With varying degrees of success, we focus on what's important and filter out the rest. This process of directing our awareness to relevant stimuli while ignoring irrelevant stimuli is called selective attention.

Selective attention is the foundation for rapid cognition, a concept made popular by Malcolm Gladwell in his best-selling book, *Blink*. When you can successfully select *only relevant stimuli*, you can think more quickly. You have a distinct advantage. Trained art experts can spot a fake museum piece in seconds. While the ball is still in the air, a former world-class tennis pro can predict when a player is about to double-fault. However, as Gladwell points out, selective attention gone wrong can be dangerous. Experienced police officers usually can tell the difference between fear and aggression by the facial expressions of suspected criminals. But when the officers are overexcited, as in high-speed chases or when guns have been drawn, they tend to miss these relevant cues. Unarmed men have been beaten or killed mistakenly because a high-adrenaline state impaired the selective attention of the officers pursuing them. Selective attention is an asset, but only when it's accurate—when you are in your focus zone.

Sustained Attention

Concentration, or attention span, is the ability to sustain attention to selected stimuli for an extended period of time. Sustained attention is necessary for productivity. We need concentration to overcome obstacles, outlast temptation, persevere through adversity, and become expert at anything. In Gladwell's examples, the art experts, tennis pro, and police officers trained themselves for many years to hone their selective attention. Their training required long hours of sustained attention so that they could fine-tune their selective attention.

Attention span increases as a child's brain matures. A normal attention span is three to five minutes for each year of a child's age. A two-year-old should be able to sustain attention for at least six minutes, and a child entering kindergarten should be able to concentrate for at least fifteen minutes. These times sound short when you consider that toddlers today can watch TV for hours. But the length of time a child can watch television or play a video game is *not* considered an accurate measure of normal attention span. TV is an exception.

Normal attention span is the amount of time you can sustain attention on a thought or activity you have freely selected. When you watch television, you are not selecting this activity free of other controlling influences on your brain. The rapid movement and edits of electronic images activate a powerful but often misused brain mechanism known as the orienting response (OR).

The "What Is It?" Reflex

The orienting response is a safety feature that was built into the brains of our ancestors. Although it still serves a useful purpose today, it also makes it hard to stay in your focus zone. To understand how the OR works, pretend you're a Neolithic cave dweller sitting in a circle listening intently to a tribal tale. You hear a noise in the bush behind you. You pause. What does it sound like? A rattlesnake! It's a good thing that noise caught your attention.

Your brain focused on the rustling in the bushes instead of the story because it's equipped with a bias for new sights and sounds. The faster and less predictable the new sight or sound, the stronger your orienting response will be. You weren't expecting to hear a rattlesnake, and you heard it quite suddenly. Your brain automatically decided that the rustling was more worthy of your attention than whatever came next in the story.

The Russian physiologist Sechenov first identified the orienting response in the 1850s, and Pavlov systematically studied it seventy years later. According to Pavlov, when something occurs that is novel to an organism, it stops what it's doing and "turns its sensors to the source of stimulation." In humans, the orienting response includes pupil dilation, reduced skin resistance, and a momentary drop in heart rate. In other words, our eyes open wide, our skin is more sensitive, and we feel attracted to the novelty. The body wants to receive the novel stimulus and take it in to be processed further. Pavlov called this survival response the "What is it?" reflex.

The orienting response has been an asset to hunters for thousands of years. It's saved the lives of generations of our ancestors, and it might save your life, too, when you cross a busy street or drive on a fast-moving freeway. In our distraction-saturated society, however, if left unchecked, the OR robs you of your ability to select and sustain your own attention.

The Click That Captures Your Attention

Timing is everything. If Sechenov and Pavlov were alive today, they'd make millions on Madison Avenue. No one studies the OR as adeptly as major advertisers. Capturing the OR is the grand prize of advertising, a $200 billion industry in the United States.

Writing for the *Media Literacy Review*, Gloria DeGartano suggests a simple experiment:

> In the evening with the lights low, put your head at an angle to the television (looking at a point right next to the screen). Wait for a commercial. Then try not to look. Try as hard as you can. What you will find out is that it is virtually impossible not to look. The quick change of images on the screen activates the brain's "orienting response." . . . We humans are programmed to look at abrupt changes in our visual field— even in our peripheral vision. It's part of our survival mechanism.

Commercials have the quickest edits, but all TV triggers the OR. On average, television edits occur every four seconds. This ongoing, repeated OR increases our adrenaline level without giving us a fair chance to say no. Nature intended us to experience the OR infrequently, or at least in moderation. An occasional boost of stimulation keeps you alert and in your zone. In excess, however, the OR overstimulates. Tiny spurt after tiny spurt of adrenaline pushes you out of your focus zone.

Think of the last time you sat on the couch and watched way too much television. When you finally turned the TV off, did you feel listless or easily annoyed? Next time someone in your house has settled in for several hours of nonstop television or video games, watch his mood when he gets up. Is he a little crankier than usual?

Habituation

If the TV is on a lot in your house, you may not see signs of irritability after someone gets up from watching, even if it's been a marathon sitting. Your family's brains may have built up a tolerance—called *habituation*—to a chronic state of mild overarousal while watching TV. In that case, if you want to see the difference that one sitting of too much television can make, first go camping for a week in the woods. After everyone gets through the crabbiness of TV withdrawal, you'll notice that you all feel more relaxed. Then, when you get home, after the first time someone watches too much TV, you're more likely to see a disagreeable shift in that person's mood.

Like coffee, TV is a stimulant, and we build up a tolerance for it. If you went for a week without coffee, your next big cup would give you a buzz. But when you're drinking coffee every day, you're not aware that you're habituating to it. Television works the same way. We overlook its drain on us because we accept it as normal.

The Digital Age of Distraction

Television is only one way we're bombarded by stimulation. Always-on media, constant advertising, new technologies, and the Internet deliver a continuous stream of sights and sounds, news and noise. Our orienting response is exploited everywhere, from big painted buses on busy streets to tiny logo stickers on fresh produce. Our ability to sort out irrelevant information is like an overclogged lint filter in a dryer. And like that dryer, we function at reduced efficiency because of it.

The concept of having more information than we can handle is certainly not new; people have complained about it since the invention of the printing press. In 1821, the poet Percy Bysshe Shelley lamented, "Our calculations have outrun conception; we have eaten more than we can digest." In *When Old Technologies Were New*, Carolyn Marvin observed that when the telephone was first introduced, people wanted to publish times next to their phone numbers "advising that they receive calls only at certain hours."

We have adjusted to the printing press, the industrial revolution, automobiles, telephones, and more. We will adjust to the onslaught of information aimed at our brains by rapidly developing digital technologies. Or will we?

In the last decade or so, experts across disciplines have been compiling data that document harmful symptoms of a rising tide of what scientists call "cognitive overload." We are starting to drown in a sea of unfiltered information and interruption.

Cognitive Overload

My Italian grandmother used to tell a story about a farmer who owned a hardworking donkey. The man wondered if the donkey would keep working hard if he fed him half as much food. The donkey did. The man, pleased to save money, halved the donkey's rations again. The hungry little donkey still did his job. Elated with his profits, the man continued to halve the donkey's food. Then my grandmother changed her tone of voice and imitated the surprised farmer: "And just when I got him to eat nothing at all, my little donkey died!"

Although I didn't understand all the words in Italian, I got the gist of the story. I've remembered it many times when I have been in situations where the more I did, the more I was expected to do. Advances in technology work this way too. The more information that becomes available, the more informed you are expected to be. As our tools make us more efficient, we're expected to give them more time and brainpower than the amount of time and brainpower they save. E-mail, instant messaging, and cell phones create pressure to make you respond. Before these technologies took over, were you expected to interrupt your own train of thought on demand?

Like the little donkey, the brain, a physical structure, has limits that cannot be exceeded. Too much information and too many interruptions deplete brain chemicals that take time and rest to replenish. As Stever Robbins warns in Harvard Business School's *Working Knowledge,* "You'll quietly lose your relaxation and recharge time, sacrificed to the gods of efficiency." Like the little donkey, you may continue to work hard. But without replenishment, you'll pay the price: cognitive overload and a harmful state of overarousal.

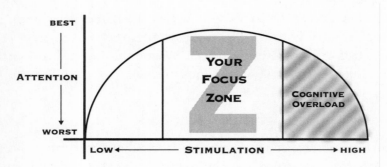

Cognitive Overload on the Upside-Down U Curve

Overwhelmed by more information than you can handle, pressured to shift gears with each interruption, you overload your circuits. Your brain tries to conserve energy by slowing down thought processing and decision making. Sometimes, a circuit breaker trips and temporarily shuts those circuits completely: you can no longer focus or make even one more decision. Or you might blow a fuse and lose your temper. In any event, you're far from being in your focus zone where your attention is at its best.

When was the last time you were working under a deadline to complete a job and things started to get away from you? Maybe the job turned out to require a lot more work than you expected, or you realized that you needed skills you didn't have. The more you used your own personal time, the more your family felt abandoned and sought you out. With all the interruptions, you got even less done. When you felt you couldn't handle even one more thing, you were experiencing cognitive overload.

When we're in this state of being overwhelmed, with no relief in sight, our stress levels surge. Our brains sense danger because, deep down, we all know how the little donkey story ends. We pump more adrenaline and remain in a state of overdrive too high to concentrate. With less focus, we get even more overwhelmed by unfiltered information and constant interruption, which create even more cognitive overload. This self-perpetuating cycle of overstimulation causes distraction, poor judgment, and social tension. It keeps us from having the attention we need to catch up on our work and break the cycle. In Chapter 10, you'll learn what you can do to carry a manageable cognitive load, even under pressure.

Boredom—Now More Than Ever

Cognitive overload—or overstimulation—is not the only problem endemic to the digital age of distraction. Boredom—or understimulation—is too, and here's why.

Years ago when Walter Cronkite reported the evening news, he was a "talking head" anchor who captivated his audience by reading full-length news stories. Now we watch rapid-fire headlines with highly graphic visuals and a moving marquee of late-breaking news that scrolls across the bottom of the screen. Since 1965, the average news sound bite has shrunk from forty-two seconds to just eight. A broadcast like Cronkite's would put us to sleep today.

In Cronkite's time, a death on a TV drama made us pause and feel sad. Then came grisly crime shows on all the major networks, sensationalized violence on the news, and casual killing in popular video games. Now a prime-time drama seems frivolous if someone *doesn't* die. In one analysis of 400 program hours of TV from 1998 to 2002, the frequency of death and violence had increased in every time slot. In one hour of prime time, blood was 141 percent more frequent and incidents of violence rose 134.4 percent. In 1998 the most common form of TV violence was fistfights or martial arts. In 2002 it was guns or weapons.

Years ago, sexy used to mean that a woman wore a low-cut dress or a tight pair of jeans. Then came the bikinis of *Baywatch*, the erotic images of music videos, and the seminudity of Victoria's

45

Secret ads. We are now desensitized to screen images and giant bill-boards that two decades ago would have seemed highly sexually provocative.

Today, one-hour reruns from the 1960s are usually cut by nine minutes to make room for added commercials. While the typical TV ad has shrunk from sixty to fifteen seconds, these highly edited commercials come in longer blocks and interrupt shows with greater frequency. Now, the length of time a program runs before commercial interruption is no longer than eight minutes and some-times only one minute, conditioning our attention to follow a story line for just a brief spurt of time.

A generation ago, sitting still was pretty easy to do. Patience and quiet listening were common for people of all ages. Today mouse clicks, remote controls, and MTV have sped up the tempo we expect from life. As Arthur Schlesinger Jr. observed, "Television has spread the habit of instant reaction and stimulated the hope of instant results."

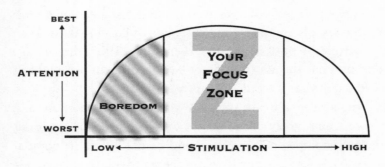

Boredom on the Upside-Down Curve

"Jolts per minute" is a measure used by screenwriters, developers of video games, and advertisers. A jolt is the jarring moment of excitement generated by a laugh, a sexy look, an act of violence, a car chase, or a quick film cut. A jolt is intended to capture your ori-enting response, by livening up the action on your screen. Jolts are creative techniques in the hands of responsible writers, producers, and marketers. But the lucrative entertainment and advertising industries have revved up both jolts per minute and jolt intensity to an extreme, abusing the orienting response and habituating us to being jolted. As media compete for your attention, these ever-increasing jolts per minute make you bored and unfocused when you have less. You need bigger and stronger jolts, or else you get stuck on the low end of the upside-down U, without enough stim to be in your focus zone.

We All Crave Adrenaline

Inside our brain, how does this occur? The brain chemical that creates the jolt in the first place is adrenaline. Action movies, fireworks, glitter, rock music, incoming e-mail at a boring meeting . . . Adrenaline makes us feel alive! We are seekers of stimulation for good reason. Stimulation makes us smarter and moves us faster so we can survive and prosper. But we need to jolt ourselves in moderation, because as we habituate to jolts, our brains build up a tolerance for adrenaline.

This tolerance occurs at the receptor site—the tiny gap between the neurons in the brain where connections called synapses take place. Biologists call this process "down-regulation." The more a receptor cell for the orienting response is stimulated, the less responsive it gets. Then we need more of the same stimulation to get just as pumped, and without it, we feel bored and restless.

Because habituation occurs inside the brain at the unseen level of the receptor site, we need to be careful not to let it fool us. The brain will think up all kinds of excuses to get more adrenaline. Just as addicts deny their addiction, we have a hidden motive to block out awareness of our growing dependence on overstimulation. "Not me," we say, but no one is immune. We each differ in our potential to develop tolerance; some brains build it more quickly than others. But habituation to adrenaline is part of our biology—a physical reality we cannot change.

Building tolerance or habituating to adrenaline can be a good or a bad thing. Habituation is useful when you want to overcome a personal fear. The more you make yourself face it, the less adrenaline you pump each time you do. Let's say you're afraid of public speaking. If you join Toastmasters and take the podium every week or two, your fear decreases a little every time. Your brain habituates to the cues—sights and sounds—that occur when you face an audience. The most effective treatments for phobias and anxiety disorders are "exposure" therapies. With support, you systematically expose yourself to your irrational fear and your brain habituates to it until it's no longer a problem for you.

On the other hand, habituation can be harmful, too. Stimulants give you a boost, but there's a price to pay. Too many lattes give you the jitters and insomnia. Too much TV causes passivity and lost potential. You need to be able to make reasonable, informed decisions. But when the brain habituates to being hyper, it quits trying to tell you what the correct price is. This puts you at risk for spending more than it's actually worth to you.

Habituating without Realizing It

Author and attention expert Thom Hartmann describes a striking example of habituation that occurred when he lived in Germany. On the autobahn, where there was no speed limit, Hartmann drove at a thrilling 110 miles per hour, amazed at cars passing him going 150 miles per hour. But a stretch of about twenty miles through a forest pass had a speed limit of 100 kilometers (roughly 60 miles) per hour. In Hartmann's words:

> It was unbearable. I felt like I was trapped, impatient and fidgety, pushing right to the edge of the 60 mph as I anticipated the end of the speed-zone and the resumption of the (literally) gas-pedal-to-the-floor speeds.

Driving at NASCAR racing speeds had conditioned Hartmann to be bored when he was driving at a speed that actually exceeds the limits on most ordinary roads.

Boredom in the Real World

Every schoolteacher today knows that boredom has become epidemic. A teacher faces an almost insurmountable challenge: having to hold kids' attention with fewer jolts per minute than kids get from 24/7 media, electronic games, and the Internet.

Kids are constantly too understimulated to perform well in their classrooms—and then overstimulated by fear of failure, because they can't make themselves pay attention to get good grades. They ride attention swings from one end of the upside-down U curve to the other.

We all battle boredom every day. We get bored with our own lives because daily reality does not deliver the jolts per minute that Hollywood reality does. We feel restless, impatient, and understimulated, wishing we could drive at 110 miles per hour all the time. Virtual worlds make our own world seem dull by comparison. In the real world, at ten o'clock tonight, you and I are far more likely to be folding laundry than solving a homicide, flying to Paris, or kissing a superstar.

Understanding why boredom is endemic to our culture helps us fight its demotivating effects. In Chapter 4 you'll learn how our culture and our choices are actually changing our brains.

What Are We Doing to Our Brains?

Neurons that fire together, wire together.
—Donald O. Hebb, PhD

The most sophisticated super-computer in the world is a Tinkertoy compared to the miracle of the human brain. The brain consists of about 100 billion neurons, and each neuron knows exactly what to do. Amazingly, every brain is a work in progress. It continues to make new connections—called synapses—in response to the choices you make every day.

Your Brain Is Changing Right Now

Brain neurons connect with each other at an astonishing rate. The adult brain has 100 to 1000 *trillion* synapses. For a long time scientists believed that the adult brain was incapable of change. New discoveries in the past fifty years have proven that view to be false. "Plasticity"—the term for the ability of the brain to change—occurs throughout life. Although the brain is more plastic in childhood, neurons continue to make new connections, form new pathways, and rewire the brain in adulthood as well. It's never too late to reshape your brain.

Plasticity is a result of what we practice day to day.

- Brain imaging using magnetic resonance images (MRIs) show that over time, as new taxi drivers learned their way around London, they enlarged the part of their brains responsible for navigation.
- The brain recordings of accomplished musicians—even those who learned to play as adults—show much more brain territory dedicated to the fingers they use to play than is true for nonmusicians.
- MRIs show that Buddhist monks who meditate daily enlarge brain regions for thoughtfulness and reflection.

Because of the adult brain's plasticity, you want to choose carefully what you practice and learn. Your habits are going down on your permanent record—your brain. It's customary to think that the brain influences behavior, not the other way around. But your brain shapes your behavior and *your behavior shapes your brain*.

As the Neuron Fires, the Brain Rewires

It takes time and practice to reshape the brain and that is a good thing. We wouldn't want our every thought, word, and deed to make noticeable changes on our permanent records. The beginning signs of brain plasticity appear to require a little less than a month. When nonmusicians learned and practiced a new sequence of finger movements, fMRIs (functional MRIs that can be done while a person moves) showed changes in brain activity patterns within three to four weeks.

For meaningful change to occur, however, brain plasticity takes a much longer time. The London cab drivers navigated around the city all day on their jobs for two years. The accomplished string players practiced routinely from seven to seventeen years. And the Buddhist monks practiced from 10,000 to 50,000 hours over a period of fifteen to forty years.

Sustained attention is necessary for brain plasticity that results from learning to occur. The London cab drivers, the accomplished string players, and the Buddhist monks sustained their attention for many hours to practice their skills every day. *Repeated practice is how we sculpt our brains, and repeated practice requires sustained attention for extended periods of time.*

Use It or Lose It

Attention shapes the brain from the very start. A human infant is born with 200 billion neurons—twice the number she will have as an adult—and immediately starts to lose the neurons she doesn't use. Remarkable as it seems, at birth every infant can clearly distinguish every phoneme of every language. Then, as infants hear only the sounds of their own native tongue, they lose the ability to process the sounds they don't need. This early natural trimming of unused neurons is called pruning.

Throughout the life span, "use it or lose it" remains true for synapses, pathways, and even entire regions of the brain. When blind people learn braille, the brain region that corresponds to their fingertips gets larger and takes over parts of the brain that would have been used for vision.

In accord with brain plasticity, the synapses and pathways that we use get stronger, and those we don't use get weaker. Ask anyone (except a math teacher) who has tried to help an eleventh-grader with a trigonometry problem. Pathways such as the meanings of sine, cosine, and tangent fade away from disuse.

Like muscles, thinking skills strengthen with exercise and weaken without it. But unlike muscles, thoughts are not visible. A glance in the mirror warns you when you're getting out of shape. In the brain, weak synapses aren't as easy to notice.

The dangers of the digital age include incessant work demands, high stress, feeling rushed, no time for intimacy, lost family time—the problems we see every day. But *the most overlooked danger of digital-age distraction may be the unseen weakening of pathways for sustained attention in the prefrontal lobe of the brain.*

YOU CAN CHOOSE WHICH BRAIN CONNECTIONS YOU STRENGTHEN

The CEO of the Brain

The prefrontal lobe is the newest part of the brain, located behind your forehead. It's the most recent development in the brain, more complex in humans than in any other animal. In a human being, the prefrontal lobe does not fully mature until about age twenty-five, and it's the part of the brain that's the most vulnerable to aging.

The prefrontal lobe is the seat of "executive functions"—the brain's CEO. It's the center for attention, planning, structuring, logic, information processing, abstract reasoning, and decision making.

Your CEO Is Busy Right Now

The prefrontal lobe is the part of the brain you use when you multitask. Actually, it doesn't let you do two things simultaneously; it rapidly toggles from one task to the other. When you e-mail, check your schedule, and listen to your phone messages all at once, your prefrontal lobe quickly switches your attention from computer to PDA to cell phone and back again. This speedy activity is fueled by dopamine, an activating brain chemical in the adrenaline family. Multitasking makes us feel sharp and creates an up-tempo feeling of getting things done. Our CEO is productive and we feel alive!

Is Your CEO Too Busy to Listen?

When you're multitasking on your computer, PDA, and cell phone, what *aren't* you doing? You aren't sitting in quiet contemplation, spending time in nature, or connecting with someone you love. These activities generate serotonin, the brain chemical linked to a sense of well-being that keeps your adrenaline brain chemicals in check. The prefrontal lobe—your brain's CEO—is rich in receptors for serotonin as well as dopamine. It's the brain region that's activated when you practice meditation, the quintessential act of sustained attention.

In one study, MRIs showed that prefrontal lobes were thicker in twenty adults who meditated routinely than in comparable controls. Increased thickness of the prefrontal lobes is considered to be a sign of resilience to stress and aging. This study was considered hopeful, because subjects were ordinary people focusing on their breathing unlike former MRI studies of Buddhist monks who had dedicated their lives to the practice. According to the report, these western subjects meditated for "only about 40 minutes a day."

When I first read about this study, I remember thinking, "*Only* forty minutes? Who has forty serene minutes a day?" Yet forty minutes a day of some kind of relaxed, sustained attention is probably the minimum you need to offset the frenzy of a workday filled with multitasking. In this digital age of distraction, our prefrontal lobes need serotonin-mediated calm and quiet to prevent being taken over by the adrenaline we pump in the course of a day.

If we could take just one serotonin moment to stop and think, we might ask ourselves what kind of prefrontal brain do we want? Doesn't a CEO need time for reflective thought? What kind of decision maker doesn't slow down, step back, and consider what's going on?

Is Your CEO Making Good Decisions?

When you're multitasking and your prefrontal lobe is switching you back and forth between tasks, are you actually more efficient?

To test this question, researchers at the Federal Aviation Agency (FAA) and the University of Michigan conducted a series of studies. Young adults multitasked math problems and recognition of geometric shapes. The problems ranged in levels of difficulty and familiarity. Results showed that in every condition, multitasking took more time than doing the problems separately. As you might expect, the subjects lost less efficiency when they were doing the simpler, more familiar tasks. But even on the simplest, most familiar problems, undivided attention was faster than divided attention.

Another study at Carnegie Mellon University found similar results and also looked at subjects' *f*MRIs. Young adults performed language comprehension tasks and at the same time mentally rotated pairs of three-dimensional figures. While accuracy did not suffer, speed did. It took longer to complete the tasks than if they had been done one after the other. Also, the amount of brain activation in the corresponding language and spatial regions was less for multitasking than for sustained attention while doing each task alone.

Findings of reduced efficiency fit with the fact that when multitasking, the brain has to shift gears each time the prefrontal lobe rapidly toggles between tasks. First, it has to choose a task; this is called "goal-shifting." Then it has to turn off the rules of the old task and turn on the rules of the new one; this is called "rule activation."

Why then do we multitask when it's actually less efficient? Well, possibly when it comes to extremely easy and familiar everyday chores, we *are* more efficient. I don't know of any studies that show reduced efficiency for emptying the dishwasher while you're on the phone.

But what about more complex tasks, when we use our computers or PDAs? The most probable answer is the immediate, uplifting effect of the activating, adrenaline-based brain chemical, dopamine. Multitasking gives you a boost of dopamine that makes you feel so alert and alive that it seems as if you're doing more in less time, even if you're not. Picture the upside-down U curve. For repetitive tasks, the cost in efficiency is small change compared to the cost of understimulation and not feeling motivated enough to stay focused. Bored and uninspired—as the digital age habituates us to be—we'd get even less done overall if it weren't for that dopamine surge.

Mindful multitasking—the strategic use of adding or subtracting stimulation as needed—requires a brain CEO that can make good judgment calls. In Chapter 5, you'll learn guidelines with helpful examples of mindful multitasking. There's a time to multitask and a time to stop. If your CEO is running on empty, the added stim of multitasking is a plus. But if your CEO is too busy, caught in a dopamine-dominant frenzy, you'll neglect to rebalance your brain chemicals with serotonin-generating downtime and you'll lose more than your efficiency. Your brain connections for sustained attention will weaken, and over time, it will get harder for you to sit still, concentrate on a problem, or patiently learn a skill.

Choosing Attention

In the digital age, we go faster, do more at once, and splinter our attention the way a prism scatters light, because we want to keep up with everyone else. But it's time to take charge and protect the brain pathways that are necessary to sustain attention.

When I was a kid, a friend's family owned some property a few blocks from the beach. His dad was a good guy and let everyone walk through his land to take a shortcut. Over time, though, he discovered that, according to the law, he had lost his ownership of the path that cut through his land. Well-meaning as he was, he suffered a loss of valuable property without realizing it. Like the shortcut to the beach, brain pathways get claimed by their daily users over time.

Based on what we currently know about brain plasticity:

- *If you're inside your zone as a habit, you're strengthening the attention pathways that you need to stay in your zone and learn.*
- *If you're outside your zone as a habit, you're weakening the attention pathways that you need to stay in your zone and learn.*

Part II gives you the tools you need to strengthen the attention pathways in your brain. You'll learn eight sets of keys to build skills and strategies to find your focus zone and stay there.

Part II

The Eight Keychains

In Part II, you'll find eight keychains of keys to get inside your focus zone. Each keychain contains key concepts and strategies to build emotional, mental, and behavior skills.

The sets of keys to *emotional* skills are:

Keychain 1 ⚷ Self-Awareness (Chapter 5)

Keychain 2 ⚷ Change of State (Chapter 5)

Keychain 3 ⚷ Procrastination Busters (Chapter 6)

Keychain 4 ⚷ Anti-Anxiety (Chapter 6)

Keychain 5 ⚷ Intensity Control (Chapter 6)

The sets of keys to *mental* skills are:

Keychain 6 ⚷ Motivate Yourself (Chapter 7)

Keychain 7 ⚷ Stay on Track (Chapter 8)

The set of keys to *behavior* skills is:

Keychain 8 ⚷ Healthy Habits (Chapter 9)

You'll find a great deal of overlap between emotional and mental skills. This reflects the reality that brain pathways for feelings and thoughts are intricately interconnected. It's effective to build your emotional skills first, though, because activation, stimulation, and adrenaline are linked to the older, emotional parts of the brain.

Each keychain has three keys, and you'll want to read about each one. Then it's time to choose your favorites and practice using them consistently. You'll find that a few trusty psychological skills and strategies will keep you focused from morning to night. They'll become the keys you want to have with you at all times, as essential as the keys to your house and car. You can then put your other keys away for safekeeping, the way you'd keep keys you don't ordinarily need every day.

As you try each key out for yourself, decide which ones unlock success for you. Use them to put together your own personal keychain to stay in your focus zone.

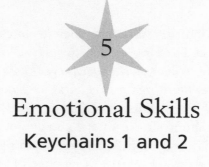

5

Emotional Skills
Keychains 1 and 2

*In a sense we have two brains, two minds—and two
different kinds of intelligence: rational and emotional.
How we do in life is determined by both—it is not just IQ,
but emotional intelligence that matters.*

—DANIEL GOLEMAN

Do you use a PDA, personal assistance software, or an agenda book but still feel disorganized or just can't keep up? Do the demands, distractions, and overload of daily life leave you grumpy or make you want to run and hide? Like many of the people I've seen in my practice, you may feel as if you've tried everything. But if you hone your emotional skills first, you'll see the difference in your productivity, your mood, and your focus.

What Is an Emotional Skill?

An emotional skill is the ability to recognize your feelings and then adjust them—as much as possible—to be more helpful to you. Sometimes, feelings give you important information about your life. Other times, feelings have been conditioned into you and they interfere with your ability to stay in your focus zone. Feelings such as anxiety and guilt act like background noise, robbing you of your ability to concentrate and stick to your plans.

Most people don't try to adjust their feelings, because it feels impossible to do so. To a large extent, that's true. But feelings can be adjusted indirectly. *While you cannot change the way you feel, you can change the way you think, and that changes the way you feel.*

Let's say that every time you pull out your PDA, you feel a wave of anxiety about all the things you've got to do by tomorrow, along with a dose of guilt about the things you didn't get done today. It feels much better to let that PDA sit in a drawer, the way a bathroom scale gathers dust during the holidays. But if you train yourself to see past your avoidance, you can face your anxiety or guilt and make a plan to deal with it. You might use calming self-talk and deep breathing, write out coping statements on index cards, or tape a favorite photo of someone you love to the back of your Palm Pilot.

Today—more than ever—you need emotional skills to stay in your focus zone. High-tech tools cannot take their place. The most sophisticated PDA, pocket PC, or expensive time management system is just a pricey paperweight if you're too frustrated, impulsive, anxious, hectic, or discouraged to use it. For this reason, I've deliberately placed the chapters on emotional skills *before* the chapters on mental skills.

How Do Emotional Skills Work?

As you practice emotional skills, you create synapses between your older, feeling brain—called the limbic system—and your newer, thinking brain: the prefrontal CEO. The more synapses you create, the stronger the connection between these two powerful brain centers—your drive and your sense of reason.

For instance, every time you look at your schedule book and say to yourself, "Hey, I'm getting there," "Progress, not perfection," or "Breathe, 1-2-3," you connect calm, confident feelings with the thought of your schedule book and your schedule. The more you practice, the more you strengthen these connections in your brain. Over time, when your prefrontal CEO thinks "schedule," your limbic system automatically delivers feelings of calm self-confidence.

Your limbic system is powerful and can either help or hurt you. Connected, your limbic system is a wealthy board of trustees who fully back your prefrontal CEO. Disconnected, when high-adrenaline feelings take over, it seizes power and strips your CEO of control.

Cognitive Strategies

Most of the keys you'll learn in this book are "cognitive strategies." A cognitive strategy is the technique of replacing unhelpful thoughts with helpful ones, which can be used to replace unhelpful feelings with helpful ones.

Chapter 5 is divided into two keychains of emotional skills:

Keychain 1 ⚷ Self-Awareness—to *recognize* your emotions and level of stimulation.

Keychain 2 ⚷ Change of State—to *adjust* your emotions and level of stimulation.

Keychain 1 ⚷ Self-Awareness

⚷ Your Observer Self

⚷ Your Adrenaline Score

⚷ The "What Am I *Not* Doing Now?" Question

According to Daniel Goleman, "Self-awareness—recognizing a feeling *as it happens*—is the keystone of emotional intelligence." But self-awareness is a challenge. In our distraction-saturated world today, we can easily lose ourselves in adrenaline-fueled diversions that make us forget tough issues which, deep down, we know have to be faced. We unintentionally slip into denial and avoid uncomfortable feelings, unpleasant chores, and disagreements with others. Meanwhile, in the back of our minds, these forgotten feelings sap us of the full power of our attention. The self-awareness keychain holds three important keys: your observer self, your adrenaline score, and the "What am I *not* doing now?" question.

⚬⚞ Your Observer Self

Who are you? Look in a mirror and ask yourself this question when you feel happy. You're bright, good-looking, successful, blessed with family and friends, and your eyes are full of life. Now face that mirror when you feel glum. You're in a rut, you look old, others have more money, you're a loner, and you're gaining weight. What a difference your mood makes!

Moods are the lenses through which we see everything around us *and ourselves*. We may be looking at the world through rose-colored glasses, or through prisms that exaggerate or distort. An observer self—sometimes called "mindfulness"—is the ability to name the lens you're looking through and remind yourself what life looks like without it.

Your Observer Self Gets You Home on Time

Let's say you're working at your desk and you hear an inviting, sociable voice down the hall at the water cooler. You are just about to pop up out of your seat to join in the conversation. Instead you pause and look to your observer self.

In a matter-of-fact way, your observer self reminds you that you're bored *and* you have to finish this project today. By turning to your observer self in this moment, you've just made an important brain connection. You've connected the feeling part of your brain to the thinking part. Now your prefrontal CEO can decide—deliberately and strategically—on a plan for success. You might choose to keep working and ignore the inviting voice at the water cooler, or you might choose to get up and walk to the cooler for a short "hello" to add a timely shot of stim to your day. Either is a good decision, and both are better than the alternatives that involve no strategy: to sit there and space out while you eavesdrop, or to jump up, join in, and lose track of time. Without your observer self, you're stuck late at work to finish the project. With your observer self, you finish on time and you're home for dinner.

Long History, Many Names

An ancient Buddhist psychology, *abhidhamma*, teaches that thoughts and feelings are transitory. By calmly observing their rise and fall, appearance and disappearance, you strengthen your sense of distance and detachment from them. This practice of mindfulness has become a basis for schools of both meditation and therapy today. Instead of reacting to thoughts and feelings instantly and automatically, you see them as events of the mind to notice and consider. You are "awake in the moment."

Your observer self is mindfulness in action. Freud described it as an "evenly hovering attention" and his students named it the "observing ego." Others call it the "impartial spectator," "witness self," "detached onlooker," "neutral bystander," and "voice of objectivity." Your observer self accepts "what is" without judgment or editorial comment. It is a reliable, rational crewmate—like Spock or Data of the Starship Enterprise—an emotionally detached voice of friendly awareness.

What It's *Not*

Your observer self is *not* the inner critic that taunts Gallwey's tennis players. If you feel shamed or nagged by your inner voice, that's not your observer self. Shake it off and try again, this time without the perfectionism. Your observer self calmly sees what you think and feel, not what you "should" think and feel.

Also, your observer self is *not* the self-conscious voice of insecurity. If you constantly wonder what others think—did you say the right thing or use the wrong fork?—you miss what *you* think. Your observer self notices your internal state, not your name-brand jeans.

Stepping Back

One day, when my children were toddlers, I overheard them talking as they watched a scary part of an animated fairy tale. My younger daughter was frightened; but her older sister pointed to the top corner of the TV cabinet and said, "Look over here." She told her little sister that this is what she did when she got scared. She explained that when her eyes could see the box around the screen, then her brain knew, "It's just a movie."

Stepping back—away from the drama—is how you connect with your observer self. When you step back even slightly from your experience, you become aware of what is happening without being immersed or lost in it. Make yourself glance away and then look at the big picture. Train yourself to see through the eyes of a director; don't get locked into the role of only one actor.

To help you break the trance of being wrapped up in your own story, you can try thinking of how someone else would see you in this moment. Do you have a friend or mentor who's been honest and frank with you no matter what? When you get self-absorbed and need to step back, ask yourself, "What would _____ say about this?

Levels of Progress

As with other brain connections, the more you use your observer self, the stronger this brain pathway becomes. At first, it may be hard to connect with your observer self; but as you practice, it gets easier.

How well do you connect with your observer self when you need to? Let's say you have a budget report due, and it's only one of a stack of monotonous jobs on your desk. A coworker whom you like, but seldom get to see, drops by to ask a question. What do you do?

a. Invite him in and talk for as long as he stays. Then walk him to the elevator and keep talking until he says he's got to go.

b. Invite him in and talk for as long as he stays, knowing in the back of your mind that you have work you don't want to do.

c. Invite him in; check the clock; decide to take ten minutes to talk with him and recharge; and then, if he's not leav-

ing, tell him you've got to get back to work and stand up
to signal that it's time for him to leave.

If you answered:	Your level of progress is:	You need to:
a	Not yet self-aware or self-controlled	Make friends with your observer self right away.
b	Self-aware, but not yet self-controlled	Do more listening to your observer self.
c	Self-aware and self-controlled	Ask for a raise.

⚬⚌ Your Adrenaline Score

*On a scale of 0 to 10, where 0 is the most relaxed
you've ever been and 10 is the most tense, what number are you right now?*

This simple question lets you rate your own current level of drive.
Variations of it are commonly used in the research and treatment of
adrenaline-fueled problems such as anxiety, fear, and anger. As a
person learns to relax, you see a decrease in both scores and symptoms.

This scale was first developed in the 1950s by Dr. Joseph Wolpe.
At that time, he called it the Subjective Units of Disturbance Scale
(SUDS) because he used it to measure unwanted symptoms that dis-
turbed a person's peace of mind. When the SUDS is used for attention control, the D stands for drive or adrenaline level. Here in the
self-awareness keychain, the SUDS is called your "adrenaline score."

Your adrenaline score is your key to gauge how slow or hyper
you feel and, if necessary, guide yourself back into the relaxed-alert

state of your focus zone. Unlike Wolpe's original intent, you're not always trying to reduce your score to become as relaxed or peaceful as possible. Instead, you're trying to adjust your level of drive to find your focus zone.

If you're:	*Your goal is to:*
in overdrive	reduce your score
low on drive	raise your score
in your zone	stay there

Your adrenaline score is a simple, practical method to check in with yourself and keep an eye on your feelings and how much adrenaline you're pumping. Some people like the scale, but some find it's too full of numbers. I suggest you give it a chance, but don't get caught up in trying to be too precise. It's fine to use a Goldilocks-and-the-Three-Bears version with just three simple ratings: too high, too low, and just right.

How to Rate Yourself

To begin using the scale, decide on some anchor points that stand for the ratings 0, 5 and 10. The best anchor points are real-life memories. Here are some examples.

0   on vacation in a hammock under a tree
5   working at your desk and getting things done
10   waiting for news about a loved one after an accident

Take a moment right now, think about the most relaxed times in your life, and decide on an anchor point for 0. Then do the same for the most relaxed-alert times for 5, and also for the most tense moments for 10.

Now that you have anchor points, you can start to practice using the full scale of 0 to 10. At various times during the day, ask yourself: *What's my adrenaline score right now?* If you practice consistently, self-rating will start to come naturally. And the more often you rate the level of your drive, the more self-aware you become.

Score	Feeling	Your Anchor Point
0	Most relaxed	
5	Usually relaxed and alert	
10	Most tense	

Your Adrenaline Score and Your Focus Zone

What's your ideal adrenaline score? That depends on the demands of your job. In Chapter 1, you learned that different activities have different focus zones. For activities that require physical strength—such as boxing and football—you need lots of adrenaline to reach your focus zone. But for most activities in the digital age—crunching code, writing reports, doing detailed research—you need patience and mental skill. You need a steady mid-range level of adrenaline to go the distance in your focus zone.

Most of the time at work, you probably want a score between 3 and 7. Very low scores —0, 1, or 2—are ideal for total relaxation but too sedate for paying attention. You'd be in your zone if you were lounging by the pool, but at your desk you're nodding off. And unless you play hockey for a living, scores like 8, 9, and 10 are usually too high to be in your focus zone.

The more often you give yourself an adrenaline score, the more you'll get a sense of what's just right for each activity in your day—a 5 at your desk, a 3 at lunch, a 7 at a sales presentation. Elite athletes who use the scale determine what score is ideal for them at various intervals before and during an important competition—a 6 on their way to the venue, a 9 when they arrive, a 7 when they're halfway to the finish line. At their best performances, they take note of their scores; then they try to duplicate them in future competitions.

Estimate your adrenaline scores on a typical day, using the following chart.

ACTIVITY	USUAL SCORE	IDEAL SCORE
Driving to work		
At my desk		
On the phone		
At meetings		
Dinner at home		

Benefits of Self-Rating

Each time you give yourself an adrenaline score, you summon your observer self. As you think about rating your feelings, you start to detach from them. And as you detach, you step back and your observer self grows even stronger.

Another advantage of your adrenaline score is that it makes you see that what you're feeling is a matter of degree. This breaks up the all-or-none quality that comes with being immersed or lost in an emotion. When you're very anxious—or angry, afraid, or stressed out—it feels as if you can't stop feeling that way. But if you give yourself a number from 0 to 10 to describe how you feel, you can see the possibility of moving down the scale by just one number—of feeling a little less that way. This makes you believe it *can* happen and breaks the grip your mood has on you.

Using Pictures Instead of Numbers

Sometimes you just can't stop and think about numbers from 0 to 10. You're so overwhelmed or fired up on adrenaline that it isn't practical. Because adrenaline reroutes the flow of blood from your brain into your muscles, it doesn't leave a lot of brainpower for rating your emotions. In an extremely high adrenaline moment, your score could seem trivial and irrelevant.

That's why mental pictures work well to signal yourself when you're topping out on the scale. The best mental pictures are metaphors—like a pot of steaming hot water on a stovetop about to boil over. I've seen classroom teachers use a technique in which they quietly place a picture card of a red traffic light on the desk of a student who's getting overstimulated. This signals the student to stop, calm down, and refocus. One artist I knew used a mental picture of a painting of Mount Vesuvius to warn herself when she was about to erupt. Many athletes use the image of the upside-down U itself to picture when they are getting too far up or down the curve.

My favorite is a metaphor I heard from a successful entrepreneur who came to see me for stress management. He was also a private pilot and wanted to train himself to stay focused at all times in the cockpit. He'd done a lot of reading, had come across the SUDS scale on his own, and understood the importance of practicing self-awareness. But he couldn't deal with adding one more instrument when he flew—even a simple 0 to 10 mental rating scale.

The SUDS acronym stayed with him and, in his mind, he created a picture of a washing machine. When he started to get too tense to hold his focus, he'd see the suds in his washing machine begin to overflow. Both he and his mental washing machine were getting way too agitated! He knew he'd better calm down fast, or else his suds would spill over and make a big mess.

⚬⚯ The "What Am I *Not* Doing Now?" Question

It takes a tough observer self to recognize anxiety, because we hide it from ourselves with distraction. The "What am I *not* doing now?" question uncovers our hidden anxiety and the diversionary tactics we use to avoid it.

Avoidance is a cinch in the digital age. Distraction is everywhere. We don't have to look farther than the TV, computer, or cell phone to escape from feelings that make us uneasy. To uncover anxiety, we need to be willing to see through our own avoidance.

If you *don't* have control of what's making you anxious, distraction is a powerful way to reduce anxiety. One study found that for children awaiting surgery, playing Game Boy reduced anxiety better than mild sedatives or holding hands with their parents. But if you're anxious about something you *do* have control over—like getting a report written on time—distraction is a minus, not a plus. Unless it's a deliberate strategy to adjust your level of stimulation (like a power break, which you'll learn about later in this chapter), playing Game Boy when there's work to be done wastes your time and masks your anxiety.

The Boredom-Anxiety Connection

If the children waiting for surgery stopped playing Game Boy, they'd think about their upcoming operation. When the brain has nothing else to think about, underlying anxiety surfaces. Often, that's exactly why we keep ourselves busy—to push unpleasant feelings away. But if you need to think about your problems, staying busy to avoid them works against you, not for you.

Linda knew her finances were a mess. She'd received a substantial divorce settlement, but now more money was going out than coming in. Linda sensed she had a growing problem, but she was too busy to think about it. She was a concerned parent who volunteered at her children's school and was on the phone a lot to plan field trips and fund-raisers with the other mothers. She was also a devoted daughter who traveled to help her elderly parents, and spent long nights on the Internet researching their health problems, insurance benefits, and care. When she wasn't on the go, Linda felt restless and unfocused. Her sleep was poor, and when her physician suggested medication, she came to see me. She needed help to face her avoidance and deal with her anxiety about her ability to handle money.

The Question That Conquers Avoidance

Linda understood that avoidance had become a habit for her. She agreed to relentlessly ask herself the question: "What am I *not* doing now?"

When Linda went to her children's school, she repeated to herself, "What am I *not* doing now?" She no longer said yes automatically when asked to volunteer. With every phone call she asked herself, "What am I *not* doing? What *don't* I want to face?" Her phone calls got shorter.

Online, Linda saw a bargain airfare to the city where her parents lived, but before she clicked to reserve a flight, she forced herself to ask the question, "If I don't go, what can I do at home instead while the children are with their father?" Every time she got on the Internet, she made herself remember, "What am I *not* doing now? . . . If I wasn't doing this, could I spend the time reviewing my finances?"

Gradually Linda faced her anxiety about money. As her nervous energy surfaced, she shuddered, had guilt attacks about her avoidance, and occasionally ate every cookie and cracker in the cupboard while trying to settle down and create a budget. She made a plan to spend at least three hours each week tackling her financial problems. Soon, Linda regained her focus. She successfully controlled her avoidance, and her avoidance no longer controlled her.

Avoidance Brings Instant Relief

We live in the "age of instant"—microwavable meals, movies on demand, instant messaging. Of course we seek instant relief when we sense underlying anxiety. Instant is our way of life, and avoidance is instant. But facing anxiety honestly is *not* an easy fix. If you had an instant solution to the problem, why would you feel anxious about it?

It's useful to have skills to reduce anxiety, like the keys on the anti-anxiety keychain that you'll learn about in Chapter 6. To get herself to sit with her finances every night, Linda played soothing music, broke her tasks into small bite-size pieces, and started each evening at her desk with a change-of-state key like four-corner breathing, which you're about to learn next.

> ## Keychain 2 ⚷ Change of State
>
> ⚷ Four-Corner Breathing
>
> ⚷ Power Break
>
> ⚷ Mindful Multitasking

A fifteen-year-old gifted student got his first A in science since the fourth grade as a result of having a gifted science teacher with a practice in her class called change of state. I don't know where she got the name; athletes sometimes use the term to describe what they do to break a pattern of under- or overdrive. Apparently she used it for the same purpose in her classroom.

Here's how it worked. Every day the students took turns being responsible for thinking up an interactive way to improve everyone's mood in three minutes or less. When the tone in the room got monotonous or tense, the student of the day was called on to lead the change-of-state activity. He could tell a joke, play music, or have everyone stand up and do jumping jacks. Some kids got pretty creative—drumming, dancing, and rapping.

Change of state kept these students in the focus zone. It was a godsend for the gifted student in my practice. This exceptional hands-on learner had built his own computer from parts when he was nine years old. It was agony for him to have to write out end-of-chapter review questions about how electricity works. Change-of-state practices kept him focused on the low-stim tasks he was getting graded on. And it taught him a valuable psychological skill to use outside science class, too, anytime he needed to get back into his focus zone.

The rest of this chapter introduces you to change-of-state strategies. Like these successful science students, you can get as creative as you want. If you work at home, pack up and go to a "third office"—your local bookstore, library, or coffee shop. If you have the flexibility, alternate jobs on your to-do list: high-stim, low-stim, high-stim, etc.

The real challenge is what to do when you're stuck at your desk, and that's what I kept in mind when I chose which keys to include here. The change-of-state keychain has three versatile new keys for you: four-corner breathing, the power break, and mindful multi-tasking.

⟊ Four-Corner Breathing

Let's start with a tried-and-true key to calm yourself quickly anytime or anywhere. With four-corner breathing, you can find your rhythm whenever you get out of sync. You can use it to pick up the beat when you're spacey or settle down when you're hyper.

Here's what you do. First, look around and find something that has four corners—a picture, a window, a door, the rectangle on this page. Now, begin:

1. Look at the *upper left-hand corner* and *inhale* for the count of 4.
2. Move your gaze to the *upper right-hand corner* and *hold your breath* for a count of 4.
3. Move your gaze to the *lower right-hand corner* and *exhale* for a count of 4.
4. Move your gaze to the *lower left-hand corner*, silently say the words, "*Relax, relax, smile,*" and do just that.

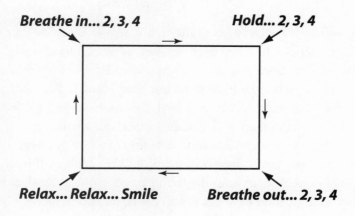

Breathe in... 2, 3, 4   Hold... 2, 3, 4

Relax... Relax... Smile   Breathe out... 2, 3, 4

Try it right now. Then use it anytime you need a quick change of pace. By gazing at a focal point outside yourself, you break up feelings of self-absorption such as worry, self-doubt, and guilt. And the practice of conscious breathing centers you and returns you to the present moment.

You can repeat the four steps over and over. If you've given yourself an adrenaline score that's higher or lower than you want, repeat four-corner breathing until you've moved at least one number in the direction you need to go. Let's say your adrenaline score is 9 and you're too tense to concentrate. Just keep doing four-corner breathing until you're at an 8.

If you already practice a breathing technique you've learned in yoga, meditation, or the martial arts, or if you've discovered that one good deep breath helps you relax and refocus, keep using those change-of-state keys, too. Four-corner breathing might still be a useful additional choice, because it combines the use of an outer focal point with inner, deep, rhythmic breathing. Women who have given birth using Lamaze methods can attest to the power of a technique that uses both.

Like versatile tools for other purposes—a measuring cup in the kitchen, duct tape in the garage, or aspirin in the medicine cabinet—four-corner breathing may become the psychological tool you reach for first when you need to refocus.

⚷ Power Break

Doug had a knack for computers but was stuck at a dead-end job. In school he had been known as an underachiever. He showed lots more promise than he delivered. When it was time to write a paper, Doug started out well enough. But when he got on the Internet to research his topic, one link led to another . . . and the paper deadline came and went.

Things weren't much different after graduation. Through a friend, Doug got a decent but dull job. He took it, thinking it would be temporary until he found a better one. But when he'd start to hunt for a new job, polish his résumé, or apply for certifications to advance himself, he got sidetracked by activities that had more pizzazz.

One day, a less talented coworker got promoted over him, and Doug decided it was time to get himself in gear. He came to see me to get tips on how to stay focused. Doug had long since figured out that he had a problem with attention. In his words, he was "drawn to distraction like iron filings to a magnet." Because of this, he'd made a rule for himself that once he sat at his desk, he wouldn't get up again until it was time to go to bed. But his plan wasn't working the way he'd hoped.

When Doug got home from the office, he was tired. He'd sit at his computer and start looking for job-related sites, but wind up surfing the net for personal interest and pleasure. His experience in school replayed itself. The deadlines he set for himself came and went. Also, more and more, he was resisting sitting down to begin at all. Straight from work, he'd go out for a beer with the guys, and then get home too late to get started.

I told Doug about the science teacher who used change of state. He said he would have been an A student in her class. He decided to adapt the practice for himself at home. He abolished his rule about not getting up and replaced it with a rule that when he needed to, he could take a strategic ten-minute-or-less break specifically to change the state he was in.

Being an inventive guy, Doug came up with a variety of breaks to rejuvenate himself—driving around the block and blasting the stereo in his car, sitting outside and watching comedy videos on his laptop, or getting on the floor and playing with his dog. He found he worked best in half-hour chunks, so that's how he timed his breaks.

Well-planned, periodic breaks gave Doug the stimulation he needed to keep working at his desk each night. He found a new job he liked, and he continued to use breaks to stay in his focus zone.

This key is called a power break because it gives you back your power to focus when you get frenzied or when you lack drive. But it also reminds you that *you have the power to start and stop your break.* To be successful at taking breaks, like Doug, you need to set a specific time to return to your work.

The Difference between Avoidance and Taking a Power Break

When I help kids to develop attention control, a pivotal moment occurs when they really grasp the difference between avoidance and taking a power break. Both avoidance and power breaks give you relief right away. But with a power break you make a commitment to return to work.

Many people get up and "intend" to get back to work, but the road to avoidance is paved with good intentions. Once you're up it's just too easy to get distracted and not go back. Doug had every intention of finding a better job but hadn't learned to control his focus so he could actually do it.

In a power break, you make a commitment—a specific promise to yourself: Before you get up, you set a time to be back. Then you keep your word to yourself the same as you would if you'd made an appointment with any other important person.

These days, with beeping alarms on cell phones, BlackBerries, PDAs, wristwatches, and computers, it's easy to set a timer. But if you can't set a timer, at least write down what time you'll return on a piece of paper. Then keep a clock nearby to check on the time. If you guess the time before you look at the clock, you might even improve your brain's ability to judge time.

If it's hard for you to return after a break, do little things to make it easier:

- Choose a task you like as the first thing to do when you get back.
- Bring a treat back with you, like a cup of tea or a pack of mints.
- Plan your next break right away to give yourself something to look forward to.

You can use power breaks to psych up, settle down, or just keep on trucking. Power breaks are good incentives to get to your next stopping place. You can plan a break at the end of each task, chapter, or section.

Tailor your power breaks to meet your own needs—lots of short breaks or just a few long ones. For low-stim jobs, you'll want to break more often. You can add mini-breaks as you need them, especially in the late afternoon. Try stretching your muscles, doing isometrics, splashing water on your face, opening a window, or turning on more lights. Novelty is a plus—even if it's just trying a new brand of sugarless chewing gum—so be creative. What's essential is that your power break is *deliberate, strategic, and time-limited*.

High or Low Stim?

To use a power break strategically, compare your actual level of stim with the level you need to be in your focus zone.

If the work you're doing is dull—repetitive data entry, technical report writing—choose a high-stim break. Do something that adds interest and energy. If you're at home, turn up your radio and sing. At the office, climb stairs while you talk to a friend on your cell phone.

If the work you're doing is nerve-racking—conflict resolution or air traffic control, for instance—choose a low-stim break to soothe and relax yourself. If you're at home, wander around your backyard or water the plants. At the office, go sit in your car or the employee lounge, close your eyes, and listen to quiet music like Pachelbel's Canon.

What if your work is both dull and nerve-racking? Let's say you're under the gun—studying for a high-stakes exam or preparing legal documents for a high-profile trial. A part of you is bored and another part feels nervous. You need a power break that's both stimulating *and* relaxing. How about going outside to be in nature and doing some light exercise?

Actually, every type of power break has some element of stimulation because novelty is stimulating. Anything you do that's different from what you're doing now can be restorative and give you a lift.

The Power Nap

At around two o'clock each afternoon, the body's circadian rhythm—its twenty-four-hour internal clock—hits a natural low. We feel sluggish and unfocused. That's why in many cultures throughout the world, people take a midday siesta.

Current research shows that afternoon naps prevent burnout. Sleep consolidates the information that the brain has recently acquired, creating more space to accept new input. Think of it like this. When you come home from grocery shopping, you put your bags on the kitchen counter and then put the groceries away. You can't fit anything else on the counter until you put the milk in the fridge, the soup in the pantry, and the ice cream in the freezer. You need to clear some counter space.

The brain works the same way. New information sits in short-term memory, waiting to get sorted into long-term storage. Burnout occurs when short-term memory—the brain's kitchen counter—is full. A relaxing break clears some space, but sometimes the counter is just too full. The brain chemicals you need to clear it—called neuro-transmitters—are too depleted. The brain's kitchen counter doesn't have room for even one more grocery sack. You need sleep to replenish those brain chemicals so they can put your brain's groceries away. An afternoon rest clears your counter—and your weary head.

You'll read more about sleep in Chapter 9. If you can't take a power nap, be sure to get plenty of good sleep at night. Sleep is nature's nightly power break so you can wake up alert, refreshed, and in your focus zone.

Vacation

Going away on vacation is your "power break of the year." A good vacation renews you and restores your perspective. On the outside looking in, you can finally see the forest; you're no longer in the middle of the trees. When you return, you're less reactive to every phone call, e-mail, or text message.

In today's competitive workplace, it's become a badge of honor to take work with you when you go on vacation. "Now there's someone headed for the top," our culture has taught us to think. But remember the starving donkey story in Chapter 3. Don't deprive yourself of the replenishment you need.

⟜ Mindful Multitasking

After a recent parent workshop, one mother told me this story. At the risk of getting mommy-tracked, she was taking time off her job as a marketing vice president to attend her son's Little League games. After one game, her son was angry at her. He had made a spectacular catch, looked up, and could tell she'd missed seeing it because she was on her cell phone. The mother got angry right back at him. How could he be mad that she'd had the bad luck to be on her phone at that very moment? Shouldn't he be grateful she was there at all, especially when she was giving up career points to do it?

When the shouting died down, they talked. He told her he really wanted her to be there, but he'd rather she not come at all if she had business to take care of. He explained that it was too hard to let go of his memory of seeing her on the phone. It would've been easier to forgive her if she wasn't there. He said that every time he remembered the play, it hurt his feelings to think she missed it. So now he didn't want to think about it at all, even though the moment had felt so good.

This conversation woke her up to her observer self. When she stepped back from her own frustration and anger, she saw what had happened in a new way through the eyes of her young son. She stopped seeing him as dramatic or spoiled and instead felt grateful to have a son who cared that much. She knew that in a few short years, he'd no longer be looking up at the stands to see her face.

This woman recognized that she couldn't concentrate on an important business call and be present for her son at the same time. She would make a different choice next time. She became a firm believer in mindful multitasking.

As you may recall from Chapter 1, mindful multitasking is the intentional, strategic practice of doing more than one thing at a time. You deliberately choose to multitask to increase your alertness, *recognizing that you're less efficient.* (Chapter 4 gave you a brief overview of this research.)

When a computer runs too many programs at a time, it processes information more slowly. The same is true for us. Like a computer, we use more internal resources when we multitask. *Mindful* multitasking takes this into account. You recognize and accept that you lose efficiency to gain alertness, but you choose it anyway because in the long run the added alertness allows you to get more done. When you can't afford reduced efficiency—when your child's faith in you is at stake, for instance—you choose not to multitask.

Be Honest with Yourself

Kyle is an exceedingly bright college student who was used to getting good grades without having to study. Recently, schoolwork started to get difficult for him, and his grades began to plummet. Kyle couldn't improvise on exams any longer. Slowly he was realizing that he had to study; but since he'd never had to before, this was hard for him to accept.

Most of his life Kyle had done his homework while watching TV. He'd habituated to having high-stim background noise. In college, he watched MTV or listened to loud rock music while he studied. When he came to see me, Kyle was adamant about continuing to do this. He'd fought about this with his parents and teachers for years, and felt strongly that he was right.

I agreed with Kyle that the added stim was helping him stay pumped to get his work done. We discussed the upside-down U and what he needed to stay in his focus zone. I told Kyle that many of the students I see create playlists of upbeat music without lyrics to use specifically while studying. They choose music that adds stim but not distraction. Kyle insisted that his music was fine for him.

Stubborn as he was, Kyle had a scientific mind. I gave him copies of research articles that showed how multitasking decreases efficiency. We talked about the trade-off between using it to get pumped yet knowing that it does decrease accuracy. Kyle agreed to an experiment. He'd bring his biochemistry assignment to our next session and his playlist of hard rock. I'd bring one of African drum-ming—instrumental, no words. He'd do his work with one playlist, then with the other, and we'd compare his time and accuracy in each condition.

Kyle arrived at the next session with no assignment and no music, but no argument either. He'd decided to run the test at home and he'd seen the difference for himself. He then created a playlist of rock guitarists such as Jeff Beck to listen to while he studied. He saved the heavy metal for his power breaks. With his new study habits, he earned back his high GPA.

It's hard to admit when the things we enjoy keep us from reach-ing our goals. Like Kyle, we're sometimes rebelling against a restric-tive voice from the past that echoes in our minds. Mindful multitasking requires maturity and making tough decisions, but the payoff is worth the effort. By deliberately choosing how to divide your attention—to add stimulation but not overshoot your mark—you remain in your focus zone with staying power for success.

Power Break or Mindful Multitasking?

When you open your e-mail program to check for incoming mes-sages, are you taking a quick break or are you multitasking? Strictly speaking, you're taking a break, even though it's usually referred to as multitasking. That's because, in point of fact, multi-tasking is actually rapid task-switching. Your brain doesn't ever truly pay conscious attention to two things at once. Whenever you multitask, you're actually taking a tiny break from one task by working momentarily on another.

The bottom line is that doesn't really matter what you call it—taking a high-speed break or multitasking. What matters is that you do it purposely and strategically, keeping in mind just the right level of stimulation you need to be in your focus zone.

Multitasking Widens the Generation Gap

When it comes to the ability to multitask, both nature and nur-ture favor young people. The prefrontal lobes of a twenty-year-old switch tasks more quickly than those of a forty-year-old, whose brain favors depth of knowledge, not breadth. Add to that the fact that most young adults today used a mouse before a crayon, and you've got a Grand Canyon–size gap between older and younger coworkers. The potential for misunderstanding about multitasking is huge.

This extra-wide generation gap is evident in most people's reactions to tiny white earbuds in the workplace. One British survey found that 22 percent of workers spend an average of three hours per day listening to MP3 players. Some managers view this as an adaptive response to open-plan office architecture. Workers used to be physically separated by walls that minimized distraction, so now they need to compensate. But other managers see it as an affront to coworkers, and they've banned MP3 players from the office. They say the headphones send a stay-away signal to others and the isolation is not good for the employee or the health of the organization. Not surprisingly, the battle lines are drawn primarily between the generations.

Multitasking, Microinequities, and Microgestures

On the other hand, damage caused by "microinequities"—minor, indirect workplace offenses—occurs on both sides of the employer-employee relationship. While managers may feel put out when workers wear earphones, workers feel demoralized when managers tell them to keep talking while they check their Treos.

These microinequities impact the bottom lines of companies that must now compete to recruit new talent to replace retiring baby boomers. As a cover story in *Time* (March 15, 2006) observed, in terms of employee retention, these slights add up to "death by a thousand paper cuts." Executives are becoming more aware of the dollar cost of the small, rude signals that multitasking can send.

Whatever your age or position at the office, when you choose to multitask, consider the value of making a "microgesture." Take a moment to tell those around you what you're doing and why.

Whether you're a worker who wants to wear earphones or a manager who needs to answer a call, see if you can send a quick signal of respect to anyone whose face you can see. You don't want to cause others to feel rejected or defensive, even if you didn't mean it. And if you're around someone who starts to multitask and it's offensive to you, speak up, but don't take it personally. Chances are you're both trying to do the same thing—the best you can in our world of distraction.

Psyching Up or Psyching Down?

If you're cleaning the garage or organizing a closet, you want all the extra stim you can get. Sip on a giant smoothie. Use a hands-free headset to yak with your buddies. Blast your favorite rock-and-roll music. You aren't at much risk of getting too stimulated to sort, stack, and recycle.

When you have serious, lengthy mental work to do, you need ways to psych up that reinforce your concentration. If you're reading tedious material, grab a fluorescent highlighter and mark up your text as you read. If you need to retain information from a dull meeting or class, take copious notes with pictures and diagrams while you listen. If every detail counts in a tiresome conversation, write everything down verbatim, as if you were a court reporter. Paper and pencil are great tools for improving your concentration.

On the other side of the upside-down U, when you're tense or hyper, you also need both physical and mental ways to calm down: relaxation exercises; a trusted friend to talk to; your favorite music and photos to soothe yourself and restore your peace of mind.

When you multitask, first make sure you know what your purpose is. Do you need to psych up or settle down? How much? You don't want to overshoot your mark. Aim for your focus zone, and choose exactly the right kind and amount of stimulation that you need to get there.

The rest of this chapter is divided into two parts: multitasking to add stim when you're low, and multitasking to relax when you're hyper.

Multitask to Psych Up

When you're bored at your desk, you need ways to add stim that keep you in your zone. Which ones might work for you?

1. *Play upbeat instrumental music.* If you're alone in your office, fiddle with the volume so it's loud enough to keep you moving, but not so loud you feel drawn to it. If you're around others and it's socially acceptable to do so, wear earphones.

Everyone has personal favorites. Go through your collection and look for instrumental music with strong rhythms and fast, steady beats. Here are some suggestions to get you started:

- *Classical*—especially lively baroque music, such as Bach's Brandenberg Concertos
- *World*—especially upbeat music featuring percussion instruments
- *Jazz*—lively, but not discordant
- *Ragtime*—how about the Scott Joplin music on the soundtrack to the movie *The Sting?*

2. *Multitask unplugged.* In the digital age of distraction, we think of multitasking as using more than one e-gadget at a time. But multitasking means doing more than one thing at a time, electronic or not. Here are some suggestions to add sensory input that is more delicious than digital.

- *Sip on something with no or low caffeine.* Mix fruit juice with water; make iced tea with herbal, white, or green tea; brew decaf coffee (which still has a little caffeine in it).
- *Munch on a healthy snack.* Cut up fruit; air pop popcorn; create your own trail mix.
- *Move your hands or feet.* Squeeze a rubber ball; rub a polished stone; point and flex your toes or rotate on the balls of your feet. Get a footrest that lets you tilt your feet back and forth. If you're alone, take off your shoes and roll a tennis ball under your feet.

3. *Connect to the digital world.* Usually this means opening a Web application—your browser, e-mail program, or instant messenger. But it can also mean text messaging, checking your PDA, or glancing at a music video you've downloaded on your iPod.

When you're sitting at your computer doing repetitive or detailed work, your connection to the Internet can feel like a lifeline. A funny e-mail or witty reply can save you from the mind-numbing effects of "terminal" boredom. Having a back-channel chat with other audience members at a lecture is now standard fare at high-tech conferences.

On the Internet you're sure to find novelty and new connections. Participatory Web sites, such as blogs, YouTube, and MySpace, invite collaboration, innovation, and social networking. You're active, not passive. It's a well of stimulation that never runs dry, which can be a plus or a minus. Chapter 10 will give you some useful tips for staying in your zone when you surf the Web. Meanwhile:

- ❏ *Go for quality.*
- ❏ *Keep a clock where you can see it.*
- ❏ *Don't let your digital connections own you.*

Multitask to Settle Down

When you're antsy at your desk, choose ways to multitask that reduce your stim so you can get back into your zone. Here are some ideas.

1. Play relaxing instrumental music. Relaxing music can sooth your soul at work, but you still need enough of a tempo to stay in your focus zone. You don't want the same music you'd select to sit in your armchair next to the fire with an adrenaline score of 1 or 2. At work, you're aiming for an adrenaline score of about 5 or 6.

For calming music, select a soft volume, just enough to hear. Again, if it's socially acceptable to do so, use earphones to create a bubble to preserve your relaxed-alert state.

As you go through your own collection, look for instrumental music that's soothing but not sedating. One guideline is to choose songs with beats per minute (bpm) for the pace you want to set. You can estimate bpm or use software such as Tangerine to analyze your music and create playlists according to bpm categories. But remember, everyone has a different threshold for adrenaline. A Chopin étude may be perfect to keep you at an adrenaline score of 5 or 6 while a nocturne puts you to sleep; the same étude may get someone else too riled up, while the nocturne puts him in his focus zone.

Here are some suggestions to get you started:

- *Classical*—try master composers such as Chopin and Beethoven.
- *Jazz*—smooth, but not elevator music.
- *Genius solo artists*—Itzhak Perlman on violin, James Galway on flute.
- *Silence*—much better than distracting noises; if it's OK with those around you, use earplugs or noise-canceling earphones.

2. *Multitask unplugged.* When you work, any kind of rhythmic breathing will help to reduce your stress. Try four-corner breathing around the edges of your computer screen. Or make a habit of taking a deep breath every time you save your work.

Little things like a pleasantly scented candle may seem too small to make a difference, yet they do. The part of the brain linked to smell is closely connected to the emotional part of the brain.

Here are more good choices:

- *Sip warm herbal tea.* Chamomile is an ancient folk favorite in many cultures.
- *Munch on a small snack of healthy comfort food.* Carbohydrates help produce soothing brain chemicals; whole-grain carbs are healthiest.
- *Tense and relax your muscles.* Tighten your fists for about ten seconds and then release and feel them relax. They'll feel warm, heavy, and tingly. The muscles in your hands are more relaxed now than they were before you tensed them. This

method is called progressive muscle relaxation, and was developed by Dr. Edmund Jacobsen more than fifty years ago. Try it one muscle group at a time, with your forehead, jaws, arms, legs, and feet. You can do it with any muscle group *except the neck*. You should never tense and relax your neck abruptly, because you could injure yourself. Sitting in chairs all day, we store tension in our shoulders. To help remedy this, tense and relax them. Hunch them up to your ears, then release; hunch them forward, then release; pull them back, then release.

3. *Take charge of your digital connections.* When you're hyper, you feel a strong pull to open new applications and start new projects. On an adrenaline rush, your brain craves more. Turn it around and recognize that in this state, less is more—less stim gives you more focus. Reduce—don't increase—your overload. Move out of your hyperalert state and into the relaxed-alert state of your focus zone.

❏ *Finish the unfinished.* Don't start another e-mail. Finish the ones you've already begun.

❏ *Stay in the here and now.* Close all the windows and applications you don't need at this moment.

❏ *Turn it into a power break.* If you just can't settle down, put your computer to sleep and go outside for a while.

Looking Ahead

Now that you've got keys to recognize and regulate your feelings, you're ready to learn even more about emotional skills. Chapter 6 covers three kinds of attention problems caused by fear: procrastination, anxiety, and varying degrees of anger. You'll get three new keychains to turn your stress into success.

Confronting Fear
and All Its Cousins
Keychains 3, 4, and 5

*We must constantly build dikes of courage
to hold back the flood of fear.*

—MARTIN LUTHER KING JR.

Nuclear threat, terrorism, global warming, pandemics, natural disasters . . . We see them up close and live on wide-screen TVs and hear them in stereo surround sound. We plant these terrifying images into our brains by watching grisly prime-time dramas and real-world horrors on the late news each night before we go to sleep.

Our brains were not built to constantly process streaming close-ups of murders, accidents, suicide bombers, disease victims, and guerrilla attacks. The orienting response (OR) described in Chapter 2 draws us in to these jolts. We need strategies to protect ourselves from larger-than-life, adrenaline all-the-time, digital-age fear.

"Fight-*and*-Flight" Causes Problems

When you feel threatened, adrenaline surges in your brain and your body. In the older, survival part of your brain, a type of adrenaline called norepinephrine triggers the fight-or-flight response, which takes many different forms today. You might experience "fight" as a feeling of anger, but it also drives anxiety, worry, and guilt—any emotion that involves irritability. When you feel disagreeable, argumentative, and oppositional, you're in a mild state of fight.

In today's world, where we often can't physically escape an annoyance or provocation, these feelings are a form of flight, too. If you're obsessively worried about the future or guilty about the past, you're also mentally fleeing from the present. When your child baits you into an argument about homework, the two of you fight and also ignore the homework that's not getting done. In fact, it might be useful to call this state "fight-*and*-flight," to make us more aware of what we're *not* doing when we're getting worked up.

Chapter 6 looks at three common problems caused by norepinephrine and the fight-*and*-flight response: procrastination, anxiety, and anger or too much intensity. It may seem odd that I use the words "anger" and "intensity" equivalently here; but it's for a good reason.

When we're provoked, our anger starts out feeling like intensity to us. People say, "I'm not angry, I'm just frustrated." Everyone around us senses anger, and later when we've cooled off, we realize how angry we sounded. But in that moment when anger is mounting inside of us, we usually think we just feel strongly about something. That's why I've chosen the word "intensity" to include all degrees of anger from fuming to furious. It will help you identify intense feelings on their way to becoming anger while you still have greater control over them.

The solutions to procrastination, anxiety, and anger or intensity begin when you see that they are, in fact, rooted in *fear*. The keys in this chapter will guide you to recognize when you feel threatened in obvious or subtle ways, and to learn methods to help you to better self-regulate your norepinephrine.

The keys you learned in Chapter 5 are also effective for the fight-*and*-flight problems described here in Chapter 6. And you'll find in this chapter—and throughout this book—that a key that comes on one keychain can also be very useful for another.

Chapter 6 gives you three keychains to keep your norepinephrine (or fear-based adrenaline) in check:

Keychain 3 ⚷ Procrastination Busters

Keychain 4 ⚷ Anti-Anxiety

Keychain 5 ⚷ Intensity Control

Keychain 3 ⚷ Procrastination Busters

⚷ Confidence Builders

⚷ Lighting the Fire

⚷ Rescripting the Past

In January 2007, Piers Steel, PhD published a study in which he analyzed hundreds of studies on procrastination. He found that procrastination is on the rise. In 1978, only about 5 percent of Americans thought of themselves as chronic procrastinators; now it's 26 percent. He also found that procrastination is strongly linked to impulsivity and distractibility, so this increased frequency made sense to him. Technology today creates greater and greater temptation to procrastinate.

Dr. Steel's analysis showed two other strong links with procrastination: your dislike for a task, which usually means that the task is low-stim; and your lack of belief that you can accomplish the task—your self-doubt, which typically is rooted in fear.

Jane Burka, PhD, another noted expert on procrastination, names three core fears of procrastinators:

1. *Fear of Failure*—If you don't do it, you won't get judged.
2. *Fear of Success*—If you do it, you'll be expected to produce more.
3. *Fear of Being Controlled*—By not doing it, you're saying, "You can't make me."

My experience with clients—and procrastination—tells me this nails it. Fear of failure includes fear of making mistakes. Most procrastinators I know have unrealistic expectations of themselves and of how things should turn out.

Fear of being controlled includes fear of speaking up for yourself. Procrastination is an indirect way to say, "I don't really want to do this." If you're afraid or feel powerless to say no, then being late, keeping someone waiting, or stalling with results becomes your way to refuse. (To break passive-aggressive habits, it's also useful to practice the assertiveness-skills key in the intensity control keychain later in this chapter.)

The procrastination busters keychain has three get-to-work keys: confidence builders, lighting the fire, and rescripting the past. Use these keys to face your own fears, stay in your focus zone, and overcome procrastination for good.

⚷ Confidence Builders

There are two main ways to build your confidence: (1) Ensure success—do things to increase your chances of getting the outcome you want. (2) Reassure yourself—define success by your efforts and value yourself whether or not you get the outcome you want.

1. Ensure Success

What happens when you play catch with a child? Instinctively, you stand close enough to the child so that she can succeed. Be the same kind of coach to yourself. In the words of Norman Vincent Peale, "Nothing is particularly hard if you divide it into small jobs."

Create goals you can achieve, and conditions so you can achieve them. Aim for progress, not perfection. Try these success builders:

- Break your job into specific steps.
- Write out a simple outline or plan.
- Include breaks and rewards after each step.
- If you're stuck, cut that step in two.
- No self-criticism; only encouragement.

If you're a pro at procrastination, become good at the "What am I *not* doing now?" question from the self-awareness keychain. Also, you'll need to call yourself on your own clever "mental self-seductions":

Catch yourself saying . . .	and counter it with . . .
"I'll do it tomorrow."	*"Now, now, now, now, now."*
"I've still got lots of time."	*"I want a margin of time to allow for the unexpected."*
"I deserve TV time."	*"I deserve to have it done now and watch TV with no guilt later."*

2. Reassure Yourself

Write down one or more of these self-statements and keep them with you, along with your simple written plan:

- Appreciate your effort. *"I give myself credit for facing this."*
- Give up being perfect. *"I like myself exactly as I am—human."*
- Remind yourself you can tolerate discomfort to reach your goal. *"I can make it." "It's tough but I'm tougher."*
- Recall a past success. *"I remember the time when I finished that _____ project well before its deadline. That felt great!"*
- Connect with your future self. *"When I'm done I'm going for a drive in the country. I can see myself now . . . relieved, happy, and free!"*
- Remind yourself that whatever the outcome, you are still a worthy person. *"Even if I get a rotten grade on this paper, I'm still intelligent and proud that I tried."*

⚷ Lighting the Fire

Since procrastination is a problem of both too much and too little stimulation, you need reliable ways to calm down when you're anxious and to psych up when you're bored. Your change-of-state keys will help. So will learning to sit down and get started when you really want to jump up and run.

Owning Your Work

Your first step is reclaiming your work as your own. Your boss, teacher, or partner may have her reasons to get the job done, but what is the core reason *you* want to do this? *"Make money," "Get a good evaluation," "Feel proud of my work," "Keep this customer happy," "Close this deal."* When you feel underpowered, repeat your reason over and over to yourself. Make it your motivational mantra. In the coming chapters, you'll learn more techniques to do this too, in the motivate-yourself and stay-on-track keychains.

Justifiable Procrastination

At the office, Greg often gets assignments by e-mail that his supervisor would not have asked for in person—writing notes after meetings, compiling details on business expenses. He stalls on completing these tasks as a way to see how important they really are. When his supervisor asks him to work on other, more immediate projects, Greg uses them as leverage. He tells his boss, "If I do this, I won't have time to get any more detailed on those expense reports."

Greg's boss thinks Greg is a procrastinator. Greg thinks of himself as a survivor. And Greg is not alone. Many workers feel forced to procrastinate as a way to control a workload that is overly demanding. With the rapid rate of change today, they often get rewarded for this behavior, because they outlast the demands that are made on them. Sensing that the company was losing interest in one of its outside consultants, Greg put off implementing the consultant's recommendations. He felt vindicated when the consultant was fired.

Using procrastination as a habit to filter out unimportant tasks can be risky, though, especially if you procrastinate outside the office too. An expert procrastinator is adept at self-sabotage. Without realizing it, you might justify your procrastination when in fact it's *not* warranted. Check in with your observer self each time you decide there's no harm in doing something later.

Planned Procrastination

Another way to use procrastination on purpose is to know when your fear of not making your deadline will kick in, and then use this knowledge to your advantage. Say you have three weeks to write a report and you can probably do it in one week. You can decide not to think about it for two weeks. Then, when you're just one week from the due date, you can use the norepinephrine from your fear of missing your deadline to get going with the report. The downside of planned procrastination is that (1) unforeseen problems can stress you out or make you late; and (2) if you do it as a habit, you condition your brain to focus only if someone imposes a deadline on you, and you lose your ability to be a self-starter.

A Shot of Fear

If you're careful, you can use a strategic shot of norepinephrine-fueled fear as a jump-start to get going. Ask yourself the question, "What is my procrastination costing me?" Make yourself name the price of your delay. Does it cause:

- Tension with yourself or others?
- Preoccupation, preventing you from doing anything else that's productive either?
- Worry about your ability to do it?
- Loss of money, such as higher prices for immediate services?
- Poor grades?
- Loss of credibility with people who matter to you?

Once you know what the bill is, face it, but don't dwell on it. Too much norepinephrine will backfire and get you stuck in a state of fight-or-flight. Think of it like lighter fuel on a fire. A little gets the fire burning; a lot makes it burn out of control.

Inspiring Quotes

In the Talmud, it is written, "A quotation at the right moment is like bread to the famished." Here is list of great starter thoughts. Check off your favorites and write them down. You can use index cards or write them on slips of paper, fortune-cookie style, and place them in strategic locations.

Which starter thoughts do you like best?

- ❑ "Start and the mind gets heated, Start and the job gets completed."—Goethe (paraphrased)
- ❑ "You don't have to be good to start, but you have to start to be good."—Mary Marshall
- ❑ "Carpe diem!" ("Seize the day!")—Horace
- ❑ "Even if you're on the right track, you'll get run over if you just sit there."—Will Rogers
- ❑ "Procrastination is the thief of time."—Edward Young
- ❑ "Just start to sing as you tackle the thing that 'cannot be done,' and you'll do it."—Edgar Albert Guest
- ❑ "Even great towers start at ground level."—Chinese proverb
- ❑ "In delay there lies no plenty."—William Shakespeare
- ❑ "You don't have to see the whole staircase, just take the first step."—Martin Luther King Jr.
- ❑ "What greater crime than loss of time."—Thomas Tusser

⌐ Rescripting the Past

Pathways in the brain hold emotional memories for a very long time. Patterns we learned in childhood during our formative years repeat themselves throughout our lives unless we recognize and change them.

Schoolchildren often feel helpless in the face of assignments and deadlines. They lack the power and maturity to protest effectively. Sometimes the only way they can say, "You can't make me," or "I don't want to do this," is to stall as long as possible. This passive-aggressive behavior annoys and provokes their parents and teachers—the authorities they seek to oppose. In this way, the child gets her desired outcome. "She's pushing my buttons," a parent might say. But from the child's perspective, she's just evening up the balance of power. Even when punished, the child still feel satisfied that her protest drew a response, so the procrastination gets rewarded, repeated, and internalized.

If you're a lifelong procrastinator, look back to the roots of your delay tactics. Did procrastination help you feel more in control as a child? Your observer self can help you out here. Remember—it's hard to see the painting when you're inside the frame.

Corrective Emotional Experience

How do you change a pattern if its pathway has been grooved into your brain? Psychologists use a method called "corrective emotional experience." In your mind, you return to the original situation, connect with the feelings you had then, only this time, you change the scenario so you think, feel, and act differently.

Chris is a freethinker who hated school as a child. Procrastination was her voice of freedom when she was growing up, but when she became an adult it interfered with her life. She was determined to stop. Both in therapy and at home, she spent time rewriting her story. She didn't blame her parents or teachers. She just imagined what it would have felt like to be given the chance to express herself and truly feel listened to as a child. She spent some time every day rehearsing this in her mind. Using the other procrastination-buster keys as well, Chris formed new habits to tackle her work, and she returned to school to complete her MBA.

Rescripting is *not* blame. Chris did not blame the adults in her life for her problems, although she was still angry at a few of her teachers. Rescripting won't work if your goal is to discharge anger.

You'll just cover the same territory over and over again, strengthening old brain pathways that you don't want. *The goal of rescripting is to build new pathways in your brain*—to form new habits that work for you. If you can't get beyond old resentments from your past, consider talking with a professional counselor.

Seeing the Past with New Eyes

Chris had a setback. One of her professors had a style that reminded her of a fourth-grade teacher whom she had strongly disliked. Intellectually, she understood that she couldn't change her professor's attitude; she could only change her own. But she resumed her procrastination.

To break the pattern, Chris rewrote her childhood scenario so that she completed assignments for her bossy fourth-grade teacher but regained her dignity in other ways. She imagined classmates supporting her and joking about this teacher, her parents validating her, and a feeling of pride that she would *not* let this teacher cause her to do anything less than her best. She soon did the same thing with her college professor, deciding that her success was more important than "showing him." This time she broke her procrastination for good.

Chris applied the self-knowledge she had gained from working with her observer self. She realized what we all need to know to resolve problems from the past: if you could go back to an old situation, you would still do all the same things you did then, because that's all you knew how to do at that time. But in your mind, you can visualize how you could have done things differently, and apply all that you've learned since that time. You *can* change.

Mental Rehearsal

To improve their skills, world-class athletes correct their past mistakes mentally and physically. I worked with a tennis player who had lost a regional title because he had missed a backhand shot under pressure. To correct his backhand error, in his mind he returned to that critical moment many times and practiced what it would have felt like to have made the shot. He pictured the position of his wrist, his line of sight with the ball, and his timing. He also imagined his emotional self in a relaxed-alert state. He visualized staying in his focus zone and withstanding the pressure of the match. He saw himself make the shot, and he made this vision even stronger than his memory of having missed it. The next year, he reached the nationals.

Brain-imaging studies show that mental rehearsal works. Remarkably, when athletes and musicians rehearse mentally, the brain activity that directs their movements is the same as when they physically perform them. Corrective mental rehearsal is accepted practice for high-level performers, and can be a powerful key for you too. You'll learn more about mental rehearsal in Chapter 7, in the stay-on-track keychain.

Keychain 4 ⊶ Anti-Anxiety

⊶ Reality Check

⊶ Make a Plan

⊶ Thought Substitution

When you want your attention to be in your control, anxiety works against you. It kicks up norepinephrine and pushes you out of your zone. Your anxiety becomes a self-fulfilling prophecy. Two well-known examples are math anxiety and test anxiety. The more you worry about getting the right answer, the more distracted you become and the less you can concentrate and get the answer right.

This happens in daily life, too. Anxiety reduces focus, and reduced focus causes anxiety. Have you ever had the experience of listening to someone, but as the person talks, you get distracted and miss what she's saying? Unsure of what you've missed, you start to feel anxious; and your anxiety, in turn, makes you even less attentive. The anti-anxiety keychain has three stay-in-charge keys to help: reality check, make a plan, and thought substitution.

⊶ Reality Check

Mary was the first in her family to go to law school. She was a hardworking student who got excellent grades. She still remembers graduation day. Her proud parents, grandparents, aunts, uncles, and cousins all came to the ceremony. A few months later, when Mary failed the bar exam, she felt as sad as she had felt happy at graduation. She had studied hard but had felt tremendous pressure while taking the exam, and she knew her anxiety was the culprit.

Mary still got a good job. In fact, her law firm was so supportive that it was paying for a tutor to help her pass the bar next time. As the test date got closer, Mary grew more and more nervous. She was biting her nails and having difficulty concentrating when she studied. Her problems absorbing the material caused her to feel even more anxious, and to wonder: Did she have the brainpower to pass this exam? A classmate referred her to me, to help deal with her anxiety.

One of the first steps I took with Mary was to look at her anxiety to see what was rational about it and what was not. Mary recognized that she was a conscientious, successful student. Although she'd always felt somewhat anxious about taking tests, she'd done well on them, even on important exams such as the LSAT to get into law school. She acknowledged that her anxiety about not being smart enough to pass the bar was irrational because it was not founded in reality. She believed that if she had enough time to study, she could master the material. But Mary had failed the bar exam once because of anxiety she couldn't control. Suppose she could not control it again? Her anxiety about her anxiety seemed rational to her. It was based in reality; it had already happened.

Rational or Irrational Fear?

The first step in fighting anxiety is to call on your observer self. Like Mary, detach and decide if you have a solid basis in reality for feeling as you do. Nature gave us norepinephrine for a reason. In

The Gift of Fear, forensic psychologist Gavin de Becker, PhD, shows how, time and again, a gnawing sense that a situation just didn't "feel right" has signaled danger and saved the lives of potential victims of violent crime.

But today, media-blitzed fear obscures authentic danger signs. We've become desensitized to our true instincts because we're bombarded by danger, disaster, and violence beamed through our living rooms and into our brains. Each night, our eyes see a basis in reality for feeling fearful even though we're safe and secure in our homes. You need a strong observer self to break this trance and disconnect from digitalized, irrational fear.

Worry feeds on itself as norepinephrine builds in the brain. The limbic system—the emotional region of the brain—makes the brain's prefrontal CEO, the thinking part of the brain, justify anxiety with thoughts that continue to produce it. Even with her law school training in logic and analytic thought, Mary's irrational fear prompted her to make unwarranted assumptions: failing the exam meant she didn't have what it took to pass; no one else in her family had gone this far in school because it was just too difficult; losing her concentration when she studied meant she had hit her intellectual limitations.

When you compare the basis of your fear with what's true in reality, you break this cycle. You insist on rational thought. Mary made herself remember her past successes. She forced herself to see that it was reasonable to assume she was smart enough to pass the exam, and unreasonable to assume she was not. The first step in dealing with anxiety, worry, guilt, or fear is to identify it as rational or irrational.

It's OK to Be Afraid

When Mary checked with her observer self about her test anxiety, she decided that this fear was rational. She might once again feel debilitating anxiety while taking the bar. She determined that the fact that she'd lost concentration in the clutch was a reasonable cause for concern. She also realized she'd been unwilling to face this before because deep down she was afraid there was nothing she could do about it. She knew how to study, but she didn't know how to get rid of her fear. By avoiding her fear, her subconscious mind was only trying to help: why let yourself dwell on things you believe you can't control? That's why it's important to give yourself a reality check and let your conscious mind decide.

Is It "Reasonable"?

In a court of law, when a case is in a gray area, the central question is: "What would a reasonable person do?" The same is true when you use the reality-check key and ask yourself, "Is this rational or irrational?" What would a reasonable person answer? After you review all the evidence, does your observer self say that your anxious feelings are an authentic message of a rational fear? Or does it say that your feelings are out of proportion to your reality? Irrational anxiety, worry, guilt, and fear usually have a grain of truth, but are greatly exaggerated. They can result from a misfiring in your brain due to culture, conditioning, or misunderstanding.

False Alarms

Dave was stunned when the paramedics told him he was having a panic attack. He felt palpitations, sweaty palms, and shakiness throughout his body and was certain it was his heart.

Panic attacks and phobias are extreme examples of irrational fear and are surprisingly common. Dave, like many others who overcome panic attacks, fought his way back to normalcy by learning to recognize that his fear was irrational. Dave learned to think of his fear as a fire alarm, a useful metaphor for any irrational, norepinephrine-fueled feelings, from mild worries to heart-pumping terror. The feelings you have are real, just as the sound of a fire alarm is real, even if there is no fire. If you lived or worked in a building where false alarms were a regular occurrence, you would learn to tolerate the awful sound of the alarm, but not feel frightened when you heard it. Dave practiced using the image of a fire alarm with no fire. He even created the image of a bunch of kids fooling around, flipping the alarm, leaving the scene, and laughing about the stupid trick they'd just pulled off. This nonthreatening mental picture broke his tension.

Irrational fear is an alarm that is broken. It sounds real, but your brain is temporarily misfiring, sending you a false alarm.

⚷ Make a Plan

Rational Anxiety

If your anxiety has a legitimate cause, make a simple, written plan for dealing with it. A good plan has three qualities: it is (1) doable, (2) specific, and (3) positive. Here's a simple test to see if you have a good plan: when you look at it, which do you feel—burdened or hopeful?

Mary's rational anxiety was her fear that feeling anxious would again interfere with her performance on the test. Once she decided to face this anxiety, Mary analyzed the reasons she had felt so anxious the first time. Like other students taking the bar exam, Mary realized that much of the pressure stemmed from its being such a public event. You don't get to pass or fail the bar in private. Everyone knows if you've made it or not. And Mary knew herself well enough to acknowledge that she was someone who dreads embarrassment because she experiences it so intensely.

Mary had been elated at graduation. She felt the family pride that had been riding on her. She realized that she had put a lot of extra pressure on herself to do well on the bar because of this. Also, her family members wanted to be supportive. They all called a day or two before the exam to wish her well. These well-meaning calls had the opposite of their intended effect, however. Mary's adrenaline went up, not down, because she felt pressured by the expectations of her well-wishers.

Mary also realized that this time, when her firm offered to pay for a tutor, she again felt a strong pressure to meet the expectations of others. She didn't want to disappoint her family or her new employers. And she felt obligated to her firm for the money it was investing in her. She was worried that her employers would think she had not been worth it.

As the test date approached, Mary started to feel more and more anxious as she studied, but this time she chose to view anxiety as an opportunity instead of a problem. It gave her the chance to practice reducing her anxiety, as she would need to do on the day of the bar. Also, she planned to use mental rehearsal when she took practice exams.

Mary decided on a three-part plan: (1) reduce pressure from others; (2) practice staying in her focus zone when she studied; (3) mentally rehearse staying in her focus zone during the exam. She wrote out a plan using keywords and phrases. A long form of it would have looked like this:

1 Reduce Pressure from Others

- Accept that it's a public event and see this as a plus, not a minus. Walk tall. Keep a paper in my pocket with the words, "I'm in the big leagues now."
- Talk with family members ahead of time, thank them for their support, tell them I'll call *after* the exam, and then screen all my calls until the exam.
- Talk with my employers and thank them for their confidence. When I think of them, think, "They believe in me. I believe in me, too."

2 Stay in My Focus Zone While Studying

- Post a giant "5" where I can see it at my desk, to remind me of the adrenaline score I want to have. Take breaks as needed.
- Put a sticker on the upper left-hand corner of my screen to remind me to practice four-corner breathing.
- Write out helpful self-talk:
  "I'm proud to be qualified to take this exam."
  "It's expensive, but not a tragedy, to have to take it again."
  "I am a test-taking animal."

3 Mentally Rehearse Staying in the Zone during the Exam

- Visualize being in the exam room at my desk getting ready to start: My heart pounds as I do four-corner breathing and say to myself, "I can do this," over and over. I settle down and focus.
- Visualize taking the test and staying in the present moment. Practice catching myself if I jump into the past with thoughts like "I should have studied more," or into the future by thinking, "I'll never make it." Use it as a cue to return immediately to the here and now. See myself pointing my finger to the place I need to look, and silently read the prompt, word for word.
- Practice these two visualizations every time I take a practice test.

Irrational Anxiety

If your anxiety does not have a legitimate cause, you'll still benefit from a simple written plan to deal with it. *Step 1* of your plan will always be the same: remind yourself it's irrational and cancel it out with a rational statement. *Step 2* will always be the same: relax. And *Step 3* will always be the same: redirect yourself to an activity that's constructive and engaging.

Mary's irrational fear was that she wasn't smart enough to pass the bar. This was her 3-step plan to deal with it:

Step 1. Write trigger thoughts and counterthoughts on an index card and keep it handy.

> Irrational: Failing the first time means I don't have what it takes to pass.
>
> *Rational: Failing the first time means I failed it the first time. Period. This actually gives me an advantage this time. I know what to expect.*

> Irrational: No one else in my family has gone this far in school, because not being sharp enough runs in the family.

Rational: No one else in my family has had the opportunities I've had. My family is plenty smart. They raised a kid who's got a law school degree.

Irrational: Losing my concentration when I study means I've hit my intellectual limitations.

Rational: Losing my concentration when I study means I'm out of my focus zone and I need to do something to get back in. Maybe it's time for a break.

Step 2. Do four-corner breathing and keep my adrenaline score below 5.

Step 3. Just keep studying. If someone else starts talking about the bar, change the subject as quickly as possible.

Mary passed the bar, and now returns to her alma mater almost every year to help others pass it too.

⚷ Thought Substitution

In the realm of the subconscious mind, forbidden fruit tastes sweet. As soon as we say no to a thought, our minds take us directly to that place. Golfers can expect to hear a splash the moment they tell themselves, "Don't go into that water trap." Instead, good golfers instruct themselves silently, "Stay straight on the fairway," and then visualize their ball sailing forward toward the green.

You cannot "not think" about something. If you're practiced at meditation, you can let a thought just "pass through." But a thought that you actively try to shut out boomerangs right back. Try it now. Don't think about cars. Whatever you do, don't think about cars. So, what kind of car are you thinking about?

In thought substitution, you get rid of an unwanted thought by trying to think about something else instead. Try this. Think about boats and bicycles and planes. Or think about a locomotive, and what it looks and sounds like as it barrels down the tracks. It's far less likely now that you're thinking about a car.

Substitutions That Work

Thought substitution clicks into place when the new thought has at least the same level of stimulation as the old one. For Mary, studying for the bar was a natural thought substitution. She substituted memorizing legal principles at the first hint that she was feeling anxious. Review questions engaged her mind and kept out thoughts of worry. As the exam got closer, she watched herself more carefully, knowing that in the time it took to wait on a check-out line at a grocery store, her idle mind could fill with thoughts of worry. She kept flash cards with her all the time, and took them out when her brain wasn't busy, even for just a few minutes.

Distraction Management

Sometimes it can be a challenge to find thoughts that are as stimulating as the thoughts you want to replace. To compete with high anxiety, you need an activity that's extremely attractive and engaging. In Chapter 5, you read about a good example of this—the study of children who played Game Boy while waiting for surgery. When these children were home working on an assignment for school, their parents wouldn't let them play a video game—it would be too distracting. But playing while waiting for surgery served a good cause: it held their attention and prevented anticipatory anxiety.

Distraction management is an intentional strategy to fight anxiety or inescapable boredom. Long-distance runners use it, imagining themselves in faraway places while their bodies conquer physical fatigue. It's not the same as avoidance or denial. Distraction management is a deliberate, conscious choice, a type of thought substitution.

Control or No Control?

Here's the most critical question in deciding whether or not to substitute a different thought or activity: *Is there anything I can do about my problem right now?* If the answer is yes, do it. Work the plan you've made, or make a new plan. When the answer is no, consider thought substitution.

The Game Boy playing children had no other options. They couldn't go anywhere or change the fact that they needed an operation. Thought substitution was their best choice.

Thought substitution, especially distraction management, is an essential psychological strategy for Olympic athletes. Consider the plight of downhill racers at the Salt Lake City games in 2002—a fairly common occurrence in the Winter Olympics. On the big day, they geared up and went up the mountain to their starting hut. There they waited for hours, not knowing if they would race or not. Finally, the judges canceled the race due to high winds. The next day, the skiers had to do it again. For hours, they sat in a small room with no windows at the top of the mountain. Sometimes they talked and laughed to break the tension. Sometimes they sat in silence. But at every moment they needed to be ready to get into their focus zone for downhill skiing and give the best performance of their life.

These skiers had mentally trained for this moment and knew exactly what thoughts would raise or lower their adrenaline scores. Sometimes, like long-distance runners, they used thought substitution and imagined being in other places at other times. This technique is also called dissociative thinking. Sometimes they centered themselves in the present moment, which is called associative thinking. Every so often, they channeled their anticipatory adrenaline into a mental rehearsal of their upcoming performance. What thoughts would you have come up with, if it had been you in that little mountain hut with nothing but your imagination to calm your nerves and keep you primed to perform?

"Engine Number 2 Is Out"

A crucial time to use thought substitution is when you're lying awake in bed the night before an exam or another major event. At this point, the critical question—"Is there anything I can do about it now?"—has only one answer: go to sleep. You need to replace your worry with sleep-inducing thoughts. But this is a huge challenge, because you can't substitute stimulating activity. The adrenaline will keep you awake. You need to rely on relaxation methods and creative approaches like this one.

Karen was a bright, hardworking woman who went back to school to get a graduate degree when she was in her mid-thirties and the mother of ten-year-old twins. With so many responsibilities in her life, she was chronically short on time to study. The night before an exam, Karen would lie awake thinking that she should have studied more. If she did fall asleep, she'd quickly wake up feeling restless and anxious.

I suggested to Karen that instead of arguing with these persistent, self-recriminating thoughts, she thank her subconscious mind for having reminded her that she could be better prepared. I asked her to reassure her subconscious mind that she got the message, and that although she agreed she could have done more, she did indeed have things under control. Then, by making peace with herself, maybe she could reduce her adrenaline and get some sleep.

Karen liked this suggestion a lot. She tried it and found that it worked. She made up a story that she could use and played it out in her mind almost every night:

I imagine I'm the captain of a ship. My first mate walks up and informs me, "Engine number 2 is out." I thank the first mate and let her know that I'm aware of the problem. I tell her the ship is safe and I'm taking care of the matter. Another crew member tells me, "Engine number 2 is out." I thank him in the same reassuring way. I remind him that we've been fine without this engine before. Several more crew members tell me about it, too. I say, "Yes, I know. Thanks for telling me," and send them away. Eventually word spreads onboard the ship. Everyone knows engine number 2 is out, and the captain can now get some sleep.

Keychain 5 ⚷ Intensity Control

⚷ Cool Off

⚷ Uncover the Fear

⚷ Assertiveness Skills

It is said that there are two good times to keep your mouth shut: when you're underwater and when you're angry. Despite this, you actually feel surer of yourself when you're mad. Not for long, though. That forceful, "I'm right" certainty is short-lived. When you cool down, you realize that yours is not the only point of view.

When you're angry, you feel like your focus is sharp. In reality, your focus is narrow and you're likely to miss important cues, particularly warning signs that you're hurting yourself or others. Anger robs you of your concentration; and left unchecked, anger perpetuates itself. The angrier you get, the more you justify your anger. And if you're arguing with someone else, anger escalates for both of you.

In *Emotional Intelligence*, Daniel Goleman coined a term that describes exactly why this is so: "amygdala takeover." The amygdala is the watchtower of the limbic system, the older, survival part of the brain. It is an almond-shaped mass of neurons whose job it is to identify danger. The amygdala reacts to all threats as if they are a matter of life or death, and hijacks the newer parts of your brain to support the fight-or-flight response. It overcomes your power of reason and forces your brain's CEO to justify your anger and create newer, better arguments to win the fight. The intensity-control keychain teaches you how to keep your brain's CEO in charge, and how to rescue it when it's held hostage during the inevitable small-scale amygdala takeovers that occur every day. The intensity-control keychain holds three keys to self-regulation: cool off, uncover the fear, and assertiveness skills.

⚷ Cool Off

Tony was a commercial real estate developer. Usually he rolled with the punches. But whenever it came time to close a big deal and tension mounted, he was quick to anger. He could not show his temper at work. But at home, he'd be irritable, bickering with his wife and flying off the handle with his teenage son. Understandably, when he was in a bad mood, they kept their distance from him. Then Tony felt abandoned and alone, just when he needed his family's support the most.

If he left the house steamed at his wife, Tony was consumed with silent rage and resentment. If he'd exploded at his son, he was preoccupied with frustration and guilt. Either way, he'd pump norepinephrine for hours at the office, impairing his ability to focus on the details of the deal he was closing.

After one particularly stormy episode, Tony's wife insisted that the family seek professional help. That's how Tony came to see me. Tony started to use his observer self right away. He learned to step back and see how pressures at work caused him to have a short fuse. He tried to keep track of his adrenaline score, but when he lost his temper, Tony still got stuck justifying his anger because he felt so right about it. As soon as he started to pump norepinephrine, all he could think was, "They've got this house and these cars and all the things they want because I do what I do. My job pays for this stuff. Couldn't they be more considerate?"

Eventually, even at his angriest, Tony came to realize that his own fear of failure, not his family's failure to understand him, was the root cause of his anger. He saw that when a big deal was at stake, with so many eggs in one basket, he felt a lot of pressure. His intensity magnified the emotional impact of anything anyone said, so it was inevitable that someone would say something that triggered his anger. Tony learned to identify his triggers—the signs of an amygdala takeover. He called it "red alert." He made a rule for himself that the moment he "saw red," he'd close his eyes, breathe deeply, and tell everyone he'd be right back. Then he would go sit in his car and listen to some music until he was "out of the red."

Apply Ice

When you get bruised, you need to stop what you're doing and put ice on your injury to reduce inflammation. This limits tissue damage. When you get bruised emotionally, the same thing happens. You become inflamed with indignity, which can cause more damage than the original injury. You need to stop and apply ice, so to speak. You need to break away from whatever's provoking you and do what it takes to cool off. This reduces emotional inflammation and limits damage—to yourself and to the people you love.

When Tony's wife said something that Tony took as a rejection, or his son did something that he felt was disrespectful, Tony got bruised emotionally. When he did not stop to cool off, Tony got inflamed and caused even more damage. He said mean things to his wife, who then felt heartbroken. He yelled at his son, who was making plans to run away. And he wrecked his own ability to stay in his focus zone at the office.

Once Tony began to "apply ice" when he got bruised, he stopped the damage from spreading. As he sat in his car listening to music, his norepinephrine quit pumping, his adrenaline score fell, and his brain's CEO took charge again. His observer self helped him see things through his wife's eyes, so that he could remember she was on his side. He also remembered what he had been like as a teen and realized that his son was just being a kid.

Stress Magnifies Emotion

Sitting in the car, Tony realized that pressure from work was the real reason he was overreacting to every emotional twitch he felt. We all overreact when we're intense because our elevated level of norepinephrine changes the way we perceive things. We experience little problems as if they were big ones, as in the story of the princess and the pea. The princess felt a tiny pea under a stack of mattresses as if it were a large lump, and it kept her awake all night. Stress amplifies emotion in just that way. You run into a tiny bump but you can't get it out of your mind. It's an obstacle until you reduce your emotional inflammation and can see your problem in its proper size.

When Tony cooled off, he quit seeing everyday misunderstandings through a magnifying lens. He also started a new habit when he left the office. If his adrenaline score was too high, he'd stop at a driving range on his way home from work and hit a pail of golf balls. That way, his adrenaline was already going down, so when he got home he could enjoy being with his wife and son, without getting thrown by the normal ups and downs of family life.

Cool-Off Tips

There's a reason why common wisdom tells you to count to ten to prevent yourself from losing your temper. Mental activity breaks the momentum of the fight-or-flight response and gets your brain's prefrontal CEO back in charge. And counting is simple enough to do even if your adrenaline is spiking. Here are some other choices along the same lines:

- Sing a song to yourself (or hum until you can think of the words).
- Clasp your hands tightly and concentrate on the tension in your fingers.
- Close your eyes and picture yourself in a favorite place outdoors in nature.
- Count backwards from 100.
- Try to remember today's date or what you had for dinner last night.

If you're having a meltdown and just can't engage the thinking part of your brain, do what Tony did: take a break and listen to music.

The fight-or-flight response sends strength to our muscles and the impulse to use them. By far and away the best temper tamer is rigorous physical exercise. Going to the driving range was a great stress buster for Tony. If you can get away from what's provoking you and go for a run or work out at a gym, you'll return more clearheaded than before, and your brain's CEO will be back in full control.

⚷ Uncover the Fear

To stop anger from recurring, you need to face the threat that triggered the fight-or-flight response in the first place. Sometimes the fear is rational and sometimes it's irrational, but it is always there, hidden underneath. *Anger is fear in disguise.*

Once you cool off, you can see your fear more clearly. It could be anything from physical danger to an old fear from junior high that you'll look silly in front of a hot girl or guy. In today's world, we all have some core fears in common.

At work, fear usually has to do with loss of money, time, status, respect, or security. Suppose your boss goes forward with a project that you don't agree with, and you're mad. Underneath, you may be afraid:

- You'll work hard but won't get your bonus.
- You're going to have to work a lot of Saturdays.
- You've lost a rung on the political ladder at the office.
- Your expertise isn't valued as it once was or should be.
- They're getting ready to outsource your job.

Deep down, angry parents fear for their child's welfare. They're afraid:

- Something harmful will happen to their child.
- Something undiagnosed is wrong with their child.
- Their child's not going to be successful.
- Their child won't be treated fairly.
- They're making mistakes as parents.

Angry couples usually fear abandonment, entrapment, or rejection. They're afraid:

113

- Their significant other is going to leave or betray them.
- They're going to be stuck in a relationship that doesn't meet their needs.
- Their significant other doesn't want them as much as they want their significant other.

Kids who are angry at their parents are usually afraid of being controlled. When they're angry at peers it's because they fear rejection, humiliation, or loss of status. At the same lightning speed that they play video games, teenagers will reject you before you can reject them. Since adolescents are constantly establishing a pecking order for popularity and dating, fear of embarrassment underlies a lot of their anger.

Other common fears that fuel anger today are being afraid of making mistakes, letting go of control, and not being good enough. Life is messy and filled with misunderstandings. If you're overly judgmental toward yourself and others, then you're also anger-prone. Deep down, you're afraid of feeling blamed, even if you yourself do the blaming.

Uncovering the fear gets your brain's CEO back in charge. As soon as you give your fear a name, your amygdala starts to let go, and you reengage the newer, front part of your brain. Unlike the amygdala, your brain's CEO sees the source of your fear as a problem to be solved, not a life-threatening event to fight or flee.

⚷ Assertiveness Skills

I was watching preschoolers being interviewed on television about events in the news. One child was asked, "Why do you think people go to war?" His reply was simple yet profound: "Because they don't use their words."

Assertiveness skills are ways to use your words so you can stand up for your rights without stepping on the rights of others. Your goal is to express yourself effectively. You don't bully others, and you don't let others bully you. Assertiveness skills help you get your needs met without passive-aggression or losing your temper. Here are some examples.

> Your boss refuses to listen to your ideas about a project.
>
> *Passive-Aggressive:* You don't say anything, but stall on getting it ready.
>
> *Hostile-Aggressive:* You blow up and quit your job.
>
> *Assertive:* You suggest a team meeting to discuss it.

> Your significant other makes plans that involve you without consulting you first.
>
> *Passive-Aggressive:* You go along with the plans but act coldly.
>
> *Hostile-Aggressive:* You blow up, slam the door, and leave.
>
> *Assertive:* You decide independently what it is you want to do. Whether or not you choose to go, you discuss the issue with your significant other.

> Your child won't turn the TV off when she's supposed to.
>
> *Passive-Aggressive:* You don't want to stop what you're doing, so you let her keep watching; but you feel resentful and snap at her the rest of the night.
>
> *Hostile-Aggressive:* You yell at her and threaten to ground her for a week.
>
> *Assertive:* You walk into the room and matter-of-factly ask her if she wants to turn the TV off or if she'd rather you turn it off; and then you follow through.

Making a Request

It's hard to use your words to solve problems when you're mad. Your amygdala is diverting your brain's resources to keep your anger burning. Your brain's CEO is less available for solving problems because the amygdala is forcing it to justify your anger and keep that norepinephrine pumping. Your focus is narrowed, and you're quicker to think, "This guy is a jerk," than "I wonder if there's another way to do this. Maybe I can talk to someone else on the team."

To help you put your words together when you feel provoked, here's a formula—a template for writing your own script:

1. *State the facts.*
2. *Say how you feel.*
3. *See through the other person's eyes.*
4. *Ask for what you want.*

Let's say you need to talk to the stubborn boss:

1. *That new software project has complications and costs not listed in the current proposal.*
2. *It's hard for me to jump on board, because I'm concerned about them.*
3. *I understand you believe it has a strong potential for success.*
4. *Let's schedule a team meeting and see what everyone else thinks.*

This time you're the frustrated parent:

1. *It's 9 pm and the TV is still on; we both know that it's time to turn it off.*
2. *I don't like having to enforce a rule you know is up to you to keep.*
3. *I know you want to keep watching and that it's been a tough day.*
4. *Do you want to turn it off or would you like me to do that for you?*

And now you're the significant other who wasn't consulted:

1. *I see you've scheduled us again to play golf with the Duffers. I'm OK with going this time.*

116

2. *I want you to know, though, that I don't like it when you say we'll go without talking with me first. I feel left out, as if I don't matter.*
3. *I know you're just trying to be sociable and plan nice things for us to do.*
4. *Next time Chip or anyone else asks you, would you say that you need to check with me first?*

Step 3 helps to defuse the situation. When you make an honest attempt to see the conflict through the other person's eyes, that person feels validated, just as you would if the other person tried to see it your way. This decreases the other person's defensiveness and also keeps the rational part of your brain in charge.

Be careful *not* to start step 4 with the word "but." With that one tiny word you change the whole sentiment of the message and undo what you said in step 3. You're no longer validating the other person's point of view. Instead you're saying, "I see your point of view, and now I'm discounting it."

Setting Limits

Technology has given us unprecedented power. With a mouse click, you can buy and sell stock, make a new friend in another hemisphere, or post an opinion for the world to see. But power comes at a price. At lectures and workshops, people have told me, "There's so much pressure today. You can't just ignore your e-mail or your cell phone," "I don't have any private time anymore," "I feel like some of my freedom has been taken away."

When someone asks, "Why didn't you answer your cell phone?" we feel that we need an excuse—"I was in a meeting," or "My battery was dead." We forget that we have the right to turn off our ringers without guilt. Having the power of technology doesn't mean we have to use it all the time.

It is necessary to draw a line. If someone "accuses" you of not answering your phone, refuse to feel that you owe that person an apology. Assertiveness skills begin with understanding and reminding yourself exactly what your rights are.

Setting limits keeps you safely in your focus zone. You're less likely to get overwhelmed and provoked to anger. Instead of tolerating interruption after interruption and blowing your stack because you can't take it anymore, you limit your interruptions to what you can handle and no more. In Chapter 10, you'll learn more tips to manage your daily interruptions. Start now to practice effective ways to say no.

You can set limits. Turn off your ringer. Screen your calls. Go offline. Put a sign on your door. If someone pops in, practice the four steps to make a request:

1. *I've got a report I need to finish.*
2. *And I'm running behind.*
3. *It's great to see you. Thanks for stopping by.*
4. *Can we catch up tomorrow? I've got to finish this and get home.*

Fear of Missing Out (FOMO)

Assertiveness means being able to say no to others, which requires you to be able to say no to yourself. When your cell phone rings, you feel a mild jolt and an impulse to action. The longer it rings, the more you fill with "fear of missing out" (FOMO).

I first became aware of FOMO while working with college students. Campuses offer a vast array of activities—lectures, concerts, enrichment classes, sports, and parties. Students can't do it all, although many make an admirable attempt to do so. The results are usually poor sleep habits, high levels of tension when papers are due, and lots of trips to the health center when burnout takes its toll. One college student in my practice even links her weight problem to FOMO. She feels that if she says no when she's offered food, she might not get the chance to taste that dish again.

You can see the fear of missing out in action when parents schedule their children for after-school activities and summer camps. I was a mom with FOMO when my children were growing up. I'd chauffeur them from soccer to dance to ceramics to swimming, hoping for green lights all the way so I could be on time. A mom with FOMO fears that other eight-year-olds have an advantage her child does not. The experts say her daughter should be playing an instrument by now, shouldn't she? And isn't the critical time for learning a second language slipping away?

Could it be that college students learned their fear of missing out from their parents? Or maybe it's an inevitable part of our fast-paced, info-rich, always-on culture today.

With so many high-stim choices available, FOMO is practically unavoidable. It lurks in the back of your mind. It keeps the remote control in your hands: what if something better is on one of your other 300 stations? It keeps you watching that ticker running across the bottom of your monitor. If stock prices change, how else can you act faster than everyone else? And it makes sure you keep track of who's online. Suppose your favorite friends have a chat and you're left out?

When you're assertive, you take charge of your FOMO. You let go of your fear that someone else is having more fun, making more money, or becoming more popular than you are. You ask yourself, "What do *I* want most?" When your cell phone rings, the only question that counts is, "Do I want to answer my phone right now?"

How to Say "No"

We all overextend ourselves. It happens for many reasons. Time is ephemeral and hard to estimate correctly. No one wants to let anybody else down or pass up an opportunity. There's FOMO, guilt, and even the habit of just plain being too nice. But you can learn and practice the art of saying no. Here are a few suggestions to get you started:

- *"I'm already overcommitted. Thanks for thinking of me."*
- *"I wish I could. It just doesn't work for me."*
- *"I'm in the middle of several projects and can't spread myself any thinner."*
- *"I'm really crunched for time. I need to pass."*
- *"My calendar is so full right now it's falling off the wall!"*

Perhaps the best-known assertiveness method is the broken-record technique. Here's how it works. Let's say the person popping into your office really wants you to take a break with him:

> Coworker: "Hey, let's go grab a frappuccino. When you get back, you'll zip through this in no time."
> You: *"No, thanks. I want to keep working now."*
>
> Coworker: "Come on. You've been slaving away. You really deserve a break."
> You: *"No, really. I want to keep working."*
>
> Coworker: "Your eyes could use some time away from that screen."
> You: *"Thanks for thinking of me. I do need to keep working."*

With the broken-record technique, less is more. You don't digress from the message. By not explaining all the details of your situation and not getting overapologetic, you streamline the communication and make it smoother for both of you.

The broken-record technique is a tool, not a weapon. Remember to stay patient and pleasant, with a tone of voice that's sincere, not rude or sarcastic. Look for an opening to shift the conversation gracefully to something that you can do instead:

> Coworker: "Hey, let's go grab a frappuccino."
> You: *"Not today. How about Friday?"* or
> You: *"I can't leave to go out, but I can walk you downstairs."*

When you emphasize an alternative, it eases the letdown of saying no—to yourself or someone else. This is actually another example of thought substitution: you purposely substitute thinking about what you can have, in place of thinking about what you cannot.

A shift away from deprivation and toward a future reward is a useful antidote to FOMO. When you need to say no to yourself, turn your attention to what you can say yes to. Try telling yourself:

- *I can't afford phone time now, but I'll call my friends this weekend.*
- *I can't take a frappuccino break now, but when I finish coding this section I'll stretch my legs and walk to the water fountain.*

Looking Ahead

You now have a range of emotional skills to practice. Chapter 7 introduces the use of mental skills. You'll learn more cognitive strategies and a new set of keys to keep yourself motivated by desire, not fear.

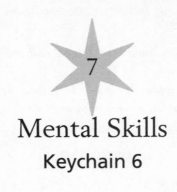

Mental Skills
Keychain 6

Nature manages to be both organized and creative.

—ANONYMOUS

I n Chapters 5 and 6, you learned emotional skills to find your focus zone when you get bored or hyper. You learned how to stop your limbic system—the older, feeling part of your brain—from taking power away from your newer, problem-solving prefrontal CEO. In Chapters 7 and 8, you'll learn *mental* skills to stay in your focus zone. You'll strengthen the abilities of your brain's CEO to cut through the demands and distractions of living in the world today.

What Is a Mental Skill?

A mental skill is the ability to use the way you think to achieve your purpose. The problem-solving prefrontal CEO is the newest, most responsive part of your brain—your leading edge. Mental skills improve powerful executive functions—decision making, planning, reasoning—which in turn lead you to success. Mental skills build with repeated practice. That's why *sustainable* motivation is critical.

The keys in this chapter are cognitive strategies—methods to help you replace unhelpful thoughts with helpful ones. The term "cognition" is taken from the Latin word *cognoscere*, which means, "to know." In psychology, cognitions refer to the many ways that the human brain can know. These abilities include perception, comprehension, learning, reasoning, and planning. Both concrete and abstract thinking are cognitions, and so is meta-reasoning, which includes beliefs, intentions, and desires.

"Hey, wait a minute," you might ask. "Aren't 'desires' feelings, not thoughts?" In fact, desires are feelings *and* thoughts. They interact in your mind as neurons interact in your brain, and this is why cognitive methods work. Although you can't change a desire directly, you can change a lot about it by changing the way you think—which is something you *can* do.

Try it out for yourself right now. Think of someone you're mad at or annoyed with—someone you know pretty well. Now make yourself think about that person's good qualities. Write them down so you can see them, and keep reading what you wrote. Visualize good times you've had together. Think about a gift this person has given you—either an actual present or something about the person that's added value to your life. Do you notice how your feelings for this person have softened a bit?

Let's consider what happened inside your brain just now as you completed this exercise. By directing attention to positive thoughts about this person, your brain's problem-solving CEO called on your emotional, limbic system to reconsider the feelings that it was linking with this individual. Your limbic system cooperated and fired more "likable" than "unlikable" pathways. You may still be miffed, but less so. Your desire for a relationship with this person is made up of both your thoughts and your feelings.

Desires are important cognitions because they sustain motivation. They do this by generating the right combination of brain chemicals to keep you in your focus zone.

Motivation by Desire, Not Fear

When you're in your focus zone, you have a balance of the brain chemicals you need to sustain your attention (which you read about in Chapter 4). You're both relaxed—pumping serotonin—and alert—pumping dopamine, with a small boost of norepinephrine.

Both dopamine and norepinephrine are kinds of adrenaline, and both sharpen your focus. (Dopamine is actually a precursor of nor-epinephrine.) But these two activating brain chemicals work very differently. Dopamine is linked with goals and rewards, and with *motivation by desire*. Norepinephrine is linked with perception of threat and *motivation by fear*. It triggers the fight-or-flight response.

A strategic shot of norepinephrine energizes you. A glimpse at a clock as your deadline approaches can spur you to work even faster. But too much norepinephrine burns you out. Although the brain has many more chemicals that interact in highly complex ways, here's a simplified guide to "brain chemistry for attention" at a glance.

	Brain Chemical		
	Serotonin	**Dopamine**	**Norepinephrine**
Function	Calms	Activates	Excites
State	Relaxed	Alert	Hyper/Intense
Thoughts	Well-being	Reward	Fight
	Cooperation	Success	Flight
	Confidence	Visions of goal	Relief from threat
Motivation	Joy of living	Desire	Fear
Type of fuel	Nourishing	Sustainable	Consuming
	Replenishes	Recycles itself	Burns out fast
To stay in your zone	Pump evenly	Pump evenly	Use sparingly

With a balance of dopamine and serotonin, and an occasional boost of norepinephrine, your brain averts fight-or-flight and you stay in your focus zone.

In this chapter, you'll learn a new set of keys—the first of two keychains of mental skills:

Keychain 6 ⚷ Motivate Yourself

These keys will help you stay *motivated by desire* and keep a healthy balance of the right brain chemicals for paying attention.

You'll have the motivation you need from start to finish—motivation you can *sustain* to pursue your goals and succeed.

Keychain 6 ⚬⚓ Motivate Yourself

⚬⚓ Goals with Meaning

⚬⚓ Sustainability Tools

⚬⚓ Deathbed Test

Achieving a long-term goal is like running a marathon. At the starting line, you're filled with enthusiasm and energy; and when the finish line is in sight, you regain focus and drive. But it's the miles in between that challenge your ability to keep running when you're tired, bored, and out of steam.

It's essential to set meaningful goals that can sustain you. Decide to run only the races you choose, the ones that matter the most to you. Then slice each goal into small, manageable pieces, to make a series of finish lines in front of you. Each time the next finish line comes into view, you'll repeatedly renew your focus and drive. That's why you want specific short-range goals—to keep one goal in sight at all times.

In *Psychology from Start to Finish*, sports psychologist Frank Schubert, PhD, says:

> The art of establishing a goal is to set it up in such a way that the task required and the rewards expected develop an irresistible power of attraction.

Here, in the motivate-yourself keychain, you'll learn how to choose goals that genuinely attract you and then set them up so they irresistibly pull you forward. Your three new keys to personal victory are: goals with meaning, sustainability tools, and the deathbed test.

⚷ Goals with Meaning

At age sixty-five, after a seven-year run in his Emmy-winning role as president of the United States on *The West Wing*, Martin Sheen enrolled in college to earn the diploma he did not get before he began his career as an actor. He certainly didn't need a college degree to boost his earning potential or increase his career opportunities. But at an age when most people spend more time thinking about tee-off times than textbooks, Mr. Sheen chose his own path for personal success. He decided on the goal that meant the most to him.

The Path with Heart

In *The Teachings of Don Juan: A Yaqui Way of Knowledge*, Carlos Castaneda gave us a pearl of Native American wisdom. Don Juan Matus, an elder shaman, is said to have advised Castaneda, "A path is only a path." You must ask, "Does this path have heart? If it does, the path is good; if it doesn't, it is of no use." The path with heart "makes for a joyful journey; as long as you follow it, you are one with it." It makes you strong, while a path with no heart weakens you.

Mythologist Joseph Campbell, PhD studied stories of human cultures around the world and throughout time. His work led him to conclude that if you "follow your bliss," doors open where before there were only walls, and where there would not be doors for anyone else. In his words:

> To find your own way is to follow your bliss. This involves analysis, watching yourself and seeing where real deep bliss is—not the quick little excitements, but real deep life-filling bliss.

In your own life, think of the difference in how you feel when you're doing something you deeply want to do, and when you're doing something that's solely an obligation. Even if you're tired, it takes far less effort to focus on work that, for you, has heart. You feel naturally motivated. But how can this apply to motivating your-self every day? Even in a job you like, much of your work is likely to be more mundane than blissful.

The Scavenger Hunt

Rob was a gifted high school junior who excelled in math and science. He had no interest whatsoever in English or social stud-ies, and his grades reflected this. Since grammar school, Rob had known that he wanted to design computer graphics for a living. He didn't see the point in studying subjects that would not help him do this. He figured that once he got to college, he'd be free of them. If he'd been aware of Dr. Campbell's advice, he would have told you he was following his bliss and counting on doors to open for him.

Rob had friends who, like himself, were skilled in program-ming and software development. They stayed in contact through high-tech interest groups on the Internet. Several were a few years older than Rob and were not accepted at the better col-leges to which they applied. Rob was shaken. The things his par-ents, teachers, and counselors had been telling him started to sink in. But Rob still couldn't motivate himself to read classics or write essays. He felt resentful and resistant.

If there was one thing Rob understood well, it was games. He had an online reputation among gamers for several tip sheets he had written for popular video games. I encouraged Rob to think of get-ting good grades as if it were a game. Instead of arguing about the relevance of what he had to do, I told him he was right. Much of the material he had to study was not going to help him in his chosen career. But getting good grades would.

We agreed that collecting good grades was a lot like a scavenger hunt. You don't really need an empty paper towel roll, a thumbtack, or last Sunday's funnies. But if you're on a scavenger hunt and these items are on your list, then you do what you need to do to get them so you can win the game.

Rob understood the analogy and changed his attitude in time to get into Cal Tech, his first choice. Since then, I've used the concept of a scavenger hunt to help many students get motivated in subjects they do not like. I've used it myself when I have to plow through paperwork that seems to have little to do with my clinical practice. It's a playful way to give yourself a shot of motivation when you're stuck with assignments that make you wonder, "What's this got to do with my job?"

Stay Connected to Your Dreams

No one's going to feel bliss every moment of the day, but you can stay connected to your sense of purpose. When Rob sat down to read a classic, he reminded himself that he was playing a game and that getting into the college of his choice was the prize. He connected the dots between his English homework and his future in computer graphics. Mentally, he drew a line between his present action and his passion, and he kept that line in mind when he sat down to work.

U.S. Olympic swimmer John Naber has won one silver and four gold medals. Naber defines motivation as "the excitement and enthusiasm you get whenever you imagine what it's going to feel like when your personal dream actually comes true." Notice the verb "imagine" in this definition. Imagining is a mental tool. When you imagine a future success that has personal meaning, you tap your dopamine-driven inner resource of *natural motivation*.

Picture a reservoir. An aqueduct leads away from it that connects directly to your house to deliver natural springwater that you can get from your faucet. The reservoir is the natural motivation you feel for your personal dream. This aqueduct is formed by the act of your imagination. You actively make yourself think of the connection between your personal dreams and what you're doing now. This gives you natural motivation on tap.

Your path with heart is unique to you. Maybe you want to make as much money as possible so you can buy a house or provide for your family. Maybe you have a particular promotion or career move in mind. Maybe, like Martin Sheen, you want to achieve a goal that you missed earlier in your life. Or maybe, like John Naber, you have a particular talent or gift and you want to see how far you can develop it. Naber says that winning Olympic medals had little or no impact on his drive as a swimmer. His dream was constant improvement, breaking his own personal best records.

Is Your Goal Worthy of Your Focus?

What is your path with heart? Where does your deep lasting bliss lie? Here are some questions to check to see that the path you're pursuing gives you the power you need to motivate yourself.

- ❑ *Is it strength-centered?* In other words, are you using the gifts and talents that you value about yourself? Does your goal make the most of your abilities and aptitudes? At the end of the day, do you feel good about your contributions?

- ❑ *Is this your own goal, or is it a result of expectations you feel from others?* Friends and family can be invaluable in supporting you and your goals, but it's easy to get caught up in "shoulds" in an effort to please others. Do you sense that others expect that you should have a certain kind of job, or go to functions or be a part of groups that don't truly interest you? People know only what you tell them about yourself. They may not know who you really are, so their expectations may not match your own path.

- ❑ *Is it believable?* It's important to be bold, think big, and be open to possibilities. It's also important to be able to sustain your own belief in fulfilling your dream. You want goals that are big enough to matter, but realistic enough to achieve. Think of going to a gym to lift weights. You add more weights only as you get stronger. If you try to lift more than you can, you'll end up hurt, discouraged, and unmotivated. In sports psychology, when you say that a goal has "maximum believability," it means that the athlete can tell you exactly how and why he can achieve that goal.

- ❑ *Do you believe in it?* Like Rob, you don't have to believe in every step of the process that gets you there. But you do need a vision that gives you a sense of purpose. Eleanor Roosevelt once said, "The future belongs to those who believe in the beauty of their dream."

❑ *Are you outgrowing it?* Our goals mature as we do. In each stage of life, we face a new inner challenge. Renowned psychologist Erik Erikson identified eight stages over the course of a life span. The first four occur before puberty. The last four are: stage 5, identity versus role confusion, in adolescence; stage 6, intimacy versus isolation, in early adulthood; stage 7, generativity versus stagnation, in middle adulthood; and stage 8, integrity versus despair, in late adulthood. What might have motivated a legend like Bill Gates to begin to transition from his role at Microsoft and become the head of a foundation to serve those in need? Most likely, he rose to answer an inner calling at a new stage in his life.

⚷ Sustainability Tools

Sustainability Tool 1: *Effort-Centered Goals*

Choose goals that depend on your efforts, not on a particular outcome you cannot control.

In 1984, Swedish psychologist Lars-Eric Unestahl turned the world of sports psychology upside down by declaring: "There is more of a chance of an athlete becoming a winner if he/she does not have winning as a goal." Dr. Unestahl had been observing world-class athletes for years to discover the habits of champions. What he found is that top athletes focus on tasks, not trophies. Their primary goal is to beat their own current level of performance, not somebody else's.

Winning the contest with yourself. When Olympian John Naber said that beating his own personal best was more important to him than winning medals, his biography backed him up. Naber didn't begin to swim until he was in the seventh grade. At first, he was the slowest swimmer on his high school team, but he enjoyed the sport. He tracked his progress with a stopwatch even when he kept losing races. He focused only on his own steady rate of self-improvement. Had he defined success by his win-loss record during this time, how likely is it that he would have continued to enjoy the sport enough to keep it up?

Competition can be a driving force for excellence. But top athletes who are fierce competitors compete first and foremost with themselves. They put personal meaning over prizes, to give themselves motivation that is sustainable. When asked, "What motivates you?" Triathlete Mark Allen, the only man to win five consecutive Ironman World Championships, answered, "Winning the Ironman or any other triathlon is icing on the cake. Realizing what I can do, going beyond what I've done before, is real success." The Ironman consists of a 2.4-mile swim across a bay, a rugged 112-mile bike ride, and a 26.2-mile marathon. Imagine the motivation you need to sustain to train for it and finish, let alone win five years in a row.

Freedom to focus on your goal. At a sports psychology conference, I was talking with a champion skeet shooter who reminded me of Dr. Unestahl's principle that winning is more likely when it is not your primary goal. He told me that when he shoots he has no idea how many clay pigeons he's already shot at. To him, the one that was just released into the sky is the only one that exists. He's focused so totally in the here and now that he's often surprised when there are no more targets left.

In addition to sustained motivation, another reason why athletes with personal goals win more is that they're free to focus completely on what they're doing in the present moment. In competition, the champion skeet shooter I met is totally engaged in each shot. When he's up, he doesn't count hits or misses to track his standing in the event. He focuses only on what he can control—his aim for the shot he is about to take.

As soon as you start to yoke yourself to someone else, you distract yourself from your own best performance. If the skeet shooter's primary goal was to win first place—to beat all the other competitors—his attention would be divided between his aim and his score. When you compare yourself with others, you wind up throwing attention away on matters you cannot control.

On any given day, you may have the best race of your life, but your competitor may have an even better one. You cannot control your competitor's performance, and if you waste your precious attention on what he's doing, you have less to give to what *you* are doing. This powerful rule applies to all human performance—sales presentations, job interviews, courtroom proceedings, public speaking, and especially taking tests.

Focusing during exams. In Chapter 6, you learned tools to overcome test anxiety. But it's best to *prevent* test anxiety by staying in your focus zone.

When you take an exam, your goal is to use every valuable moment to focus on answering questions and solving problems. The moment you start to wonder how the person next to you is doing, what your grade is going to be, or if everyone else is better prepared than you are, you're throwing good attention away. What's more, since you cannot control how well others are doing or what your percentile rank will be, you are tethering yourself to uncertainty, which creates anxiety and pushes you out of your focus zone.

If you have trouble staying focused during exams, pinpoint the warning signs when you start to lose focus:

- Looking up and seeing others working.
- Losing your place on the page.
- Thoughts such as "How come everyone else can do it and I can't?"

These are the moments when you're starting to burn too much norepinephrine. Learn to identify them immediately. On an exam, you want your brain's problem-solving CEO to stay in charge, so allow only dopamine- and serotonin-generating thoughts. Try replacement self-talk such as:

- *What matters is my own self-improvement.*
- *I'm staying in the here and now.*
- *I'm prepared to do this.*

Dealing with performance pressure. Exams and major events aren't the only times that you come face-to-face with the pressure to perform. The tension you feel when you compare yourself to others can be a problem in daily life, too.

> Carol was a sales associate who shared a large open office space with others. She was a dynamo who moved fast and worked hard all day, but hit a low in the mid-afternoon. Then, she'd sit quietly at her desk, overhear the other sales reps on their phones, and start to doubt her abilities. Why could they do more than she could? What did they have that she didn't? The rest of the afternoon became a self-fulfilling prophecy. With low self-confidence, she didn't close many sales.
>
> Usually Carol's competitive streak worked in her favor. Imagining herself winning this month's sales contest could pump her up. But in her afternoon slump, thinking about the competition made her feel worse, not better.

Because Carol pushed herself hard beginning early in the morning, her brain chemicals for paying attention were getting depleted by mid-afternoon. Sensing that she'd be running on empty soon, her brain started to pump norepinephrine. In a fight-or-flight state, Carol's fears began to grow. Her adrenaline score was too high, not too low, and thoughts of competition drove it even higher.

Carol needed to pace herself better, but she also had to deal with her mid-afternoon fear of low performance. She had to quit comparing herself unfavorably with others. She made a plan to use counterstatements: *"This is only one small slice of the day. I don't know what he was doing an hour ago." "Everyone has strong times and weak ones." "Maybe it's just his turn and mine's coming up next."*

Carol was accustomed to scripting what to say to counter a

prospect's sales resistance, so she easily caught on and quickly saw good results. Carol also wrote positive self-statements on index cards:

> *I do what I can in a day, and it's a lot.*
> *I'm refilling my fuel tanks.*
> *What I think matters, and I think I'm good.*

For years, Carol had used the phrase "eyes on the prize" to keep herself pumped and focused. She continued to use it, even when she felt low, but when she said the word "prize," she made sure that she thought only of her own personal goals.

One of the times when everyone is particularly vulnerable to performance pressure is at the start of a new job or any new situation. Without a track record, your entire self-worth seems to ride on every conversation, decision, or sale. During the first week at a new company, a new location, or a new school, you compare yourself to others almost all the time. A prominent trial attorney once told me that although he had tried multimillion-dollar cases, none caused him more angst than his very first trial. At the time, he felt as if that verdict would define him as a winner or a loser.

When you face the challenge of performance pressure, detach from the competition around you and remember who you are. Return your thoughts to your own personal goals. Picture Tiger Woods and the "block out everything except the shot" expression on his face when he's on the eighteenth green. How much of his attention is he squandering on his competitors, and how much is on the putt he's about to take?

Your own private victory. Feeling too self-conscious can cause you to choke in an important moment or an ordinary one—in a boardroom or a classroom, in front of thousands or alone at your desk. You have the choice to focus instead *only* on your own actions, to free yourself from caring about embarrassment or loss of status.

In describing his high school days, John Naber recalls that at times he was the slowest swimmer in the pool. But his personal goal—what he and his father cared about—was getting a better time than he did in his last race. He was not distracted by his public loss; he focused entirely on his private victory.

The ancient Taoist Chuangtzu wrote wistfully about an archer who has all his skill until he shoots for a prize of gold. The archer then sees two targets. His skill has not changed, but the prize divides him. He thinks more of winning than of shooting. And the need to win drains him of power.

When your goal depends on your efforts, not a prize, you'll get motivation that lasts and focus that won't be wasted on factors you can't control. Aim for self-improvement—to do your personal best.

Benchmarks. When psychologists talk about choosing goals that are based on effort, the objection usually raised is accountability: "I don't want a surgeon who is trying his hardest; I want a surgeon with a record for success." Choosing goals that are based on your personal best doesn't mean you disregard the outcome. You can still be results-driven. In fact, you are freer to accept the results as your own, and be even more responsible for them.

Let's say you're waiting in pre-op for your surgery. The patient in the operating room before you doesn't make it. Do you want a surgeon who is tied to the outcome and is still thinking about what just happened when you're wheeled in? Or do you want a surgeon who knows he did his personal and professional best, accepts the existence of factors beyond his control, and is now ready to focus fully on you and your procedure?

The surgeon who did his best knows the survival rates for the operation he just performed. Being aware of records, statistics, and benchmarks is an important part of doing your personal best. You want to take these numbers into account without letting them own you or rob you of your focus.

The business world is filled with numbers with which to measure yourself—sales quotas, earnings per quarter, target price, stock performance, return on investment. When you're beating them, it's great. But when they beat you, it's not. The challenge is to redefine these numbers as useful feedback, much the same way pilots use the feedback they get from their instruments to fly a plane. Some numbers tell you to make a course correction; most just need to be watched; a few indicate potential danger. A pilot checks his instruments, responds accordingly, and continues to fly the plane to his destination. The information guides him, but it's not the reason he flies.

Feedback is necessary for learning, and benchmarks are yardsticks so you can understand better what your feedback means. The challenge is to keep the benchmark in its proper context. Whether you make your sales quota or not, the question that helps you to make progress is: what can you learn from it?

When you get feedback, be a pilot with new information from one of your instruments in the cockpit. How does it help you fly your plane? If you're too busy worrying or being upset, you probably won't learn much, because you're out of your focus zone. But if you accept feedback for what it is, you can use it to get where you want to go.

"Reframing" is a cognitive strategy in which you change your perspective or point of view. In Chapter 8, you'll learn more about it. A benchmark is a useful servant but can be a tyrannical master. Learn to reframe your benchmarks as helpful feedback, not unhelpful threats.

Sustainability Tool 2: *Stairway to Success*

Build a set of climbable steps so you can reach your goals.

Remember that the art of establishing a goal is to set it up in such a way that each task and its reward develop an irresistible power to pull you forward. A metaphor that is used in sports psychology is to think about building a flight of stairs. You want each step to be just the right size and all the steps to be in the right order, so that each one leads to the next. As you climb, you gain the momentum you need to take you to the top.

To make the stairs sturdy enough to hold your weight, you need to define the size and shape of each step. *Specific is terrific*. Clearly state what you will accomplish and by when you will have it complete. Put this in writing to make it even more concrete.

If you're feeling overwhelmed about your work, it's likely you don't have a sturdy staircase. Imagine for a moment that you're at the construction site of a house that is just being framed. You look up and see the framing of the second-story door; but with no stairs, you have no way to get up there. If that's your assignment—to get up to the second story—you feel at a loss for what to do next. You look around but can't see how this can be done.

When a job you face starts to overwhelm you, use your feelings as a signal to build a set of stairs. Build each step big enough so you can make progress but small enough so you can expect success. The middle of a staircase is the hardest. Build in a landing—an attractive power break.

If you're struggling, resize your steps to make them smaller and easier to face. If you feel overwhelmed by that big stack of receipts to record, sort them out into two or more stacks, and then record one stack at a time.

Keep in mind your imaginary race with the series of many finish lines. As you cross each one, your next one comes into view right away. You get rewarded each time with a boost of dopamine that keeps you motivated, moving along, and in your focus zone.

Sustainability Tool 3: *Bending Tree*

Be goal-guided, not goal-governed.

Remember Tim Gallwey's "shoulds" at the beginning of Chapter 2? According to Gallwey, self-criticism is the worst enemy of focused play in tennis. It robs you of the joy of play, so you lose your motivation for the game.

In my practice I see the damage caused by unbending "shoulds" in today's world of unsustainable extremes:

- Students who get either A's or F's because they strive for perfection in the classes they like, but can't sustain the effort for the classes they don't like.
- Chronically overweight people who start out on diets that they follow to the letter, until they can't, and then they binge.

- "Clutterholics" whose desks are stacked with piles of papers, except periodically when that they are totally clear, at the start of the newest unrealistic system for keeping things in order.

We can learn a lot from Mother Nature, who is powerful and strong, yet adaptive and flexible. In nature, bendable is dependable.

You can be flexible too, by being goal-guided, not goal-governed. Instead of all-or-none thinking about your goals, bend your rules from time to time. Think of what could happen instead:

- A perfectionist student resists following every hyperlink to every reference to write the definitive work on the topic, makes time to study for a less preferred class, and gets A's, B's, or C's in all his subjects.
- A dieter goes to a party; gives himself permission to eat a reasonable portion of a dessert; and later, at home, does not feel the urge to open every cupboard and overindulge.
- A worker who feels compelled to keep every piece of paper until he can read it again and be certain what to do with it accepts the fact that if he accidentally throws away something he needs, he'll deal with it. As his workspace clears up, he discovers that he can find what he needs more easily.

Tree in a storm. When you drive yourself too hard, you burn out and feel unmotivated. Then you blame yourself, feel guilty, and drive yourself even harder. Also, you aren't prepared to withstand the inevitable setbacks you experience every day.

Picture a sturdy, well-rooted, tall tree in a storm that bends as much as it needs to, so it does not break. You can do this, too.

⚷ Deathbed Test

Although this practice may sound dark at first, the deathbed test is one of the most enlightening motivational tools I know. It's simple.

When you have to make a tough decision, ask yourself this question: "At the moment of my death, if I look back to this moment, what do I want to remember that I decided to do right now?"

You've got to be willing to imagine the moment of your death with a degree of objectivity. You don't need specifics—age, place, or cause of death. You just need that gut feeling of finality—the kind you felt when you closed the door behind you for the last time after moving your furniture from the last place you lived.

The Destination We All Share

Another legend of our times, Steve Jobs, gave the commencement address to the class of 2005 at Stanford University. Jobs, founder of Apple computers and Pixar studios, explained that at age seventeen, he read a quote that made a lasting impression on him. He said it went something like this: "If you live each day as if it were your last, some day you'll most certainly be right." Since then, for the past thirty-three years, he's looked in the mirror every morning and asked himself, "If today were the last day of my life, would I want to do what I am about to do today?" If the answer has been no for too many days, he knows that he needs to change something.

Jobs said, "Remembering that I'll be dead soon is the most important tool I've ever encountered to help me make big choices in life." He explained that external expectations, pride, and fear of embarrassment or failure "just fall away in the face of death." Then he described a close brush with death that he'd had that year, when he was diagnosed with pancreatic cancer. It turned out to be a rare form, curable by surgery, but until that was discovered, Jobs stared his own mortality in the face.

As a result, Jobs felt that he could say with even more certainty that death is "very likely the single best invention of life" because it is "life's change agent." In his words:

Death is the destination we all share. . . . Your time is limited, so don't waste it living someone else's life. . . . Have the courage to follow your heart and intuition. They somehow already know what you truly want to become.

A Thought of Death Each Day?

Albert Camus once said, "It's no use reminding yourself daily that you are mortal; it will be brought home to you soon enough." But many spiritual traditions—and Steve Jobs—disagree. They use thoughts of death for good, not gloom—as an impetus for life every day.

Another Yaqui teaching from Castaneda's Don Juan is to keep the mental picture of a black crow sitting on your left shoulder, to motivate good decision making in your life. With death so close to your head at all times, you are bound to stay focused and choose the right course of action.

Depending on how much you fear your own death, you'll kick up some norepinephrine when you use the deathbed test. As you may recall, a strategic shot of norepinephrine is energizing, but too much flips you into a state of fight-or-flight. To stay in your focus zone when you think about death, stay centered on its power to motivate, the way Steve Jobs did.

You can use the deathbed test every day or just when you need it. You can look in the mirror, imagine a crow on your shoulder, or create your own imagery. You might prefer the pleasant mental picture painted by seventeenth-century English poet Robert Herrick: "Gather ye rosebuds while ye may."

Looking Ahead

The mental skills you've learned in the motivate-yourself keychain will serve you well over time. In Chapter 8, you'll learn more mental skills, including the cognitive strategies of self-talk, reframing, and mental rehearsal. Your new keys will unlock your ability to build the structure you need to achieve your goals without adding unhelpful pressure.

Structure without Pressure
Keychain 7

(When asked what book he would choose if he were shipwrecked on a desert island): A practical guide to boat building.

—BERNARD BARUCH

To stay in your focus zone, you need structure—schedules, plans, to-do lists. Otherwise you'll feel foggy at one extreme of the upside-down U; or frenzied, at the other extreme.

Structure keeps the brain chemicals for attention pumping in a balanced way. A routine or step-by-step plan connects you to your goals so that you generate dopamine. And it reassures you so that you generate serotonin, too.

Adding a deadline can give you a strategic shot of norepinephrine, but too much pressure creates tension and kicks you into a state of fight-or-flight. You might feel a surge of sharper focus for the moment, but in the big picture you have less concentration, not more.

A good example is the situation of the well-meaning parents in Chapter 1 trying to help their distracted child settle down and do his homework. Not realizing that the child is already scared he can't do the work, the parents threaten to take away his privileges. Instead of motivating the child, the threat causes a meltdown that makes it harder, not easier, to get the homework done.

What you need in situations like these is to build structure without adding pressure. You want climbable stairs that are not too steep or scary. If you're a parent helping a child who's afraid at homework time (although he may not know or admit it), give him a safe set of steps to follow. For example, if your child is scared he can't write a good essay, read the question with him and then work together to construct a simple, step-by-step list of what he has to do next. Write it out clearly: Step 1—What's your theme? Step 2—Name three things you can say about it. Leave spelling and grammar for last so he feels that it's safe to use any word or phrase he thinks of. If your child gets stuck coming up with ideas, draw a simple picture of the sun and ask him to write the main idea in the center and something about it on each ray. If your child is afraid he can't do a math problem, write out a model solution that he can keep in front of him to follow. When you patiently create a helpful guide for your child, you remove the threat that's immobilizing him, without giving in to his fear and doing the work for him.

Structure, such as step-by-step self-instruction, is effective for any job that is new, is complex, or involves pressure, especially if you're having a problem getting started. For instance, if you have a report or presentation to prepare, list what you have to do from beginning to end. As you write it down, you might discover that one of those steps has been a hidden source of pressure for you—the reason you've been putting the whole thing off. Perhaps you need some information, but it's lost in a disorganized file cabinet or you have to contact a difficult coworker to get it. Now you can break that step into its own set of steps. The task becomes doable and the fear disappears. Methods like these provide *structure without pressure*.

This chapter gives you a second keychain of mental skills:

Keychain 7 ⚷ Stay on Track

These methods are high on structure but low on fear. In the stay-on-track keychain, you'll learn how to use three keys that you've already seen in action in previous chapters: self-talk, attitude shift, and mental rehearsal.

Self-talk includes self-instruction, like the strategies in my doctoral dissertation that you read about in the Introduction. You'll learn how to choose specific words and phrases to direct yourself to stay on task. *Attitude shift* is based on a cognitive strategy called reframing, which you read about in Chapter 7 when we reframed benchmarks as helpful feedback. *Mental rehearsal* is a type of visualization to strengthen new associations and brain pathways. In Chapter 4, you read about the effects of mental rehearsal on brain plasticity.

Keychain 7 ⚷ Stay on Track

⚷ Self-Talk

⚷ Attitude Shift

⚷ Mental Rehearsal

Some people say that they don't like structure or schedules because making plans robs them of their spontaneity. Often, this is code for "I don't want to get roped into this," or "I'm holding out to see if something better comes along." Deep down, we all know that if an event or project is important and we want it to come off smoothly, we make a plan. Builders have blueprints, directors have storyboards, and entrepreneurs have business plans. A memorable wedding, comfortable retirement, happy vacation, move to a new house, or surprise birthday party are all the results of good planning.

Written plans have power. When you see a technique you like in this keychain, *write it down*. You can use shorthand, keywords, symbols, abbreviations, or simple pictures. Index cards work well; they're portable, palm-size, and durable. Post-its are handy, too; you can slap them down almost anywhere. Or you may prefer to go paperless and post an electronic note on your computer desktop.

Why put your plan in writing? It's human nature to assume that you'll have better recall in the future than you actually do. Behavioral scientists call this principle "foresight bias"—the tendency to believe you can retrieve information just because you're familiar with it. When subjects predict what they can recall while material is in front of them, they consistently overestimate what their actual recall scores will be. (That's why it's best to overlearn when you study and quiz yourself with flash cards, not just read the material.) So, outsmart your foresight bias. Grab a pencil and paper right now. As you read this chapter, write down the strategies you plan to use.

⚬⚊ Self-Talk

In this section, you'll learn precision self-talk that is brief and to the point. I'll describe five types of self-talk to you: (1) the 3-item to-do list; (2) self-directions; (3) anchors; (4) affirmations; and (5) thought substitution (which you learned in the anti-anxiety keychain, and which has even more uses here).

1. The 3-Item To-Do List

Simplify. The first time I met Josh, he described his mind as a "complicated mess." Josh is a chemist who heads up a team that holds several patents. He has a classic "Edison trait" profile: he's an inventive individual who, like Thomas Edison, is predominantly a divergent thinker. In other words, he thinks of many things at once without the usual filters that censor out seemingly irrelevant associations. The upside of this trait is that he thinks of things no one else thinks of; the downside is that often he's thinking of them while everyone else is thinking or talking about something else.

To cope with his divergent style of thinking, Josh had trained himself to carry around a book with blank pages so he could write down his ideas and things to do. He found that once he had written them down, it wasn't as difficult for him to listen to others.

Josh told me that he was never without his list, so I was surprised when he told me it wasn't helping him get things done, because he seldom if ever looked at it. He, in turn, was surprised that I would consider the list to be useful to him as a reminder. His sole purpose was to free his mind by writing down his thoughts. When he showed his list to me, I saw why he didn't pay attention to it. At eight pages long, it was overwhelming. One task was "Apply for grant renewal"; the next was "Pick up dry cleaning."

I suggested to Josh that he choose the next three things he needed to do and write them down on a Post-it. He did, and immediately saw the benefit of this practice and developed a new system. His 3-item list was more inviting and drew him into it, instead of repelling him away from it.

Josh continued to add items to his long list, so he could relieve his mind of the burden of carrying these thoughts around in his head. But he also kept a 3-item to-do list, which gave him a dopamine-driven spurt of focus and motivation each time he used it and got something done.

Strategize. If you use a to-do list, you might notice that when you're particularly drained, you put easy things on your list to build up momentum. Don't feel silly doing this: it's an effective strategy. Go ahead and list a gimme or two—water the plants, sharpen your pencils, air out the coffeemaker. These little chores are avoidance only if they're all you do. If you use them as a warm-up, you're skillfully using a psychological tool. *Nothing succeeds like success*. You can practically feel the surge of rewarding dopamine when you cross something off your list.

Another effective strategy is to alternate high- and low-stim items. If a boring, repetitive task leaves you low on adrenaline, then your next to-do list item will supply you with more.

Have two distinct 3-item to-do lists: one for your workplace and one for home. Josh found that doing this helped him in several important ways. Since his lab work was more stimulating than his responsibilities at home, having an at-home to-do list kept him focused on his lower-stim tasks there. It also helped him leave his daytime problems at the lab so he could be more present for his wife and children at night. And by detaching from his lab problems, he could face them again with fresh eyes the next morning.

You'll find that your brain likes a short written list of just three tasks at a time. If something more urgent arises, you can *replace*, not add, an item at any time. With just three items, you cruise right along. While you're doing one task, your brain programs itself subconsciously to tackle what's coming up next.

Ready-made substitute thoughts. The 3-item to-do list is ideal for thought substitution, which you'll read about again later in this section. As you may recall from Chapter 6, thought substitution is crucial at times, because you can't make yourself *not* think about something, but you can make yourself think about something else. The next item on your to-do list is an immediate, able substitute thought. When you catch yourself having an anxious thought, feeling bored, or getting distracted, replace that unhelpful thought with the next item on your to-do list.

Let's say the first task on your 3-item to-do list is to finish writing a report summary. As you settle in at your desk, you start to feel anxious about your annual performance review coming up this Thursday. Your mind cycles through a checklist of things you've done right and wrong this past year, and you hear yourself defending your less wonderful decisions to your invisible supervisor. You start to wonder where you've placed files you might need to explain your decisions, and you fight the urge to search for memos about updates on review procedures. You can't "not think" about the review, but you can substitute the thought "report summary" and repeat it to yourself over and over again, as you guide yourself back on track.

When Josh had to relocate because of his job and was in the midst of his move, he was on the verge of feeling overwhelmed most of the time. He was selling one home and buying another, moving everything he owned, helping his wife and children adjust, reorganizing his new workspace, and dealing with the politics in his lab. When he started to feel anxious or fearful, he refocused on whatever was next on his 3-item to-do list. He learned to prevent feeling overwhelmed by substituting that one precise self-instruction each time his mind wandered or froze. Then he silently repeated it to himself until he was back in his focus zone.

2. Self-Directions

Josh used the next item on his to-do list as an effective *self-direction*—the practice of silently telling yourself what to do *right now.* Probably you've already used this method. Have you ever walked from one room to another to get something and forgotten what you went there to get? When you figure it out, if you're like most people, you say it over and over again to yourself until you walk back with it in your hands.

Self-direction calls you back to your immediate situation. It's a trusty substitute thought if you're getting distracted. Like Josh, you can make yourself recall the next task on your 3-item to-do list. By repeating it as a steady self-command—or a simple keyword like the name of the item you needed from the next room—you replace the thoughts, such as daydreams, urges, or anxieties, that are distracting you.

In today's world, self-direction is especially useful for setting boundaries between work and personal life. Josh used self-direction to remind him to stick with his work to-do list when he was at the lab, and to shift to his home to-do list when he walked through the door. As he drove down the driveway, he repeated a simple reminder: *"I'm home, home, home, home, home, home."*

The self-talk I taught my subjects for my doctoral dissertation was self-direction. Some subjects used the sentence *"I will do my work"* or repeated, *"Work, work, work, work, work, work."* The subjects who silently said, *"No, I will not listen,"* or its short form, *"No,"* were using a technique called "thought-stopping" in which redirection is implied. In thought-stopping, you train yourself to use the word "no" as a signal to return immediately to what you were doing. Another variation is to wear a rubber band around your wrist and snap it as you say the word "no" to direct yourself back to work.

Use "do," not "don't." If you say to yourself, "Don't dawdle," your subconscious mind hears "dawdle." Instead say, "Let's go," or "Move it."

Here are some all-purpose self-directions to help you stay in your focus zone. Check the ones you like best, and add some of your own:

❑ *Focus*

❑ *Pay attention*

❑ *Concentrate*

❑ *Keep working*

❑ *Stay alert*

❑ _____

❑ _____

Concise verbs that are specific to what you're doing are powerful self-directions, because by naming the action, your brain has already begun to take you there. For example:

If you're . . .	Say . . .
Drafting a technical report	*"Think, write, think, write, think, write."*
Creating a spreadsheet	*"Keep it straight; be accurate."*
Meeting a future deadline	*"Pick up the pace; keep moving."*

3. Anchors

An anchor is a concise word, phrase, or image that grounds you, just as an actual anchor keeps a ship from drifting off to sea. Verbal anchors are short, simple, and easy to recall.

Although most anchors are present-tense, here-and-now thoughts, some connect with past and future events to anchor you to the feeling, mood, or energy level that you need in the present moment. For example, by remembering a past success, you anchor yourself to your belief in yourself, so you can go forward with confidence. In the section on mental rehearsal, you'll learn to include anchors when you rehearse. That way, when you use them later, they'll connect you back to the skills you practiced during your mental rehearsal.

Vary your use of anchors. That way, they'll stay novel and keep their dopamine punch. The anchors I'll cover here are goals and tasks; past success; supportive people; and mood.

Goals and tasks as anchors. You've already been introduced to goals as anchors, when you learned to repeat a personal goal over and over to yourself to overcome procrastination. When you repeat the next item on your to-do list, or when you remind yourself concisely of what you need to do next, you're using a task as an anchor. Actually, a task is a goal: it's your most immediate one.

You can use the name of any type of goal—long-term, intermediate, short-term, immediate—as an anchor. For example:

Long-term: MBA

Intermediate: bachelor's degree in economics

Short-term: A in macroeconomics

Immediate: Study this chapter

Go ahead and make your goals into anchors by giving each one a name. If you'd like, you can go back and review the goals-with-meaning and stairway-to-success keys in Chapter 7 to help you do this.

Long-term: _____

Intermediate: _____

Short-term: _____

Immediate: _____

Past success as an anchor. Most of us are much better at remembering past mistakes than past successes. We constantly replay the demoralizing nagging of our inner critic. Instead, we need to hear encouraging messages from within—the voice of an inner coach who anchors us to our strengths and skills.

Make yourself remember at least three successes that have personal meaning for you. If you can, recall successes that are relevant in some way to your immediate task. For example, if you're preparing for an important presentation, think of the last time you successfully stood in front of others to talk.

Now write down three past successes to use as anchors:

Success 1: _____

Success 2: _____

Success 3: _____

Does one of these successes evoke particularly strong self-confidence for you? If so, find a photo, keepsake, or souvenir that you can use as a touchstone to anchor you to this memory and use it to boost your morale.

Supportive people as anchors. At the University of Wisconsin, experiments found that flashing the names of selected friends and relatives motivated subjects to work harder at tasks of verbal fluency, analytic reasoning, and functional creativity. These rapid reminders of loved ones boosted the subjects' persistence on these tasks, which required concentration and problem-solving skills. The positive results held even when the names were flashed for just a fraction of a second.

Interestingly, only names of friends and relatives who subjects said shared their goals or supported them in their goals resulted in improved scores. Names of those who regarded the subjects' goals as unimportant had the opposite result. In those cases flashing the name reduced task persistence.

These results agree with what I've seen in my practice. We all think about other people a lot. But do we think about the right people at the right times?

Who believes in you? Here are some typical answers I've heard through the years:

- "My mom and dad always thought I could do it."
- "I had a teacher in college who made me feel like I was smart."
- "My kids make me feel like I can do anything."

Next time you're unsure of yourself, and you picture your boss firing you, or see yourself standing before an imaginary judge defending your actions in a courtroom, substitute thoughts of the people who believe in you. Like the subjects in the University of Washington study, you'll get a boost in your concentration and problem-solving skills.

Jeff was a college student whose father died of cancer. He became preoccupied with his grief and lost his ability to concentrate. He was at risk for failing out of school, and decided to fight back with cognitive strategies. He had a black belt in karate, and from his experience in the martial arts, he knew how powerful psychological tools could be.

Jeff began using cognitive strategies right away. With time and deliberation, he made an entire deck of index cards. On each card he wrote one or more self-statements, to counter each of the distracting thoughts he had, especially his fears about the future. He wrote: "My mother is healthy and will probably live a long time" . . . "I can get a good job and support myself" . . . "I can handle money."

Despite her own grief, Jeff's mother was immensely supportive of him. She encouraged him to practice with his cards. Slowly but surely, Jeff fought and won back his focus and his success at school.

Jeff kept one card in his pocket at all times—his ace in the hole for any occasion. He'd made several copies of it, which he had laminated. But it wouldn't have mattered if he had lost the card. Jeff knew every word by heart. It had served him well many, many times, when nothing else could get him back on track. On this card he had written:

My Mom believes in me.
My Dad believes in me.
And I believe in me.
I can do it.
I hold the power.

Borrowing someone else's belief in you when you need it is like standing at a cash register, ready to pay for what you're buying, when you discover you don't have enough money. Then someone gives you the difference between the price that's just been rung up and what you have in your wallet. And you don't have to pay that person back. You already have—by your effort to live up to the belief that the person placed in you.

Take a moment right now and write down the names or initials of three people, living or dead, who are on your side:

1. _____

2. _____

3. _____

The next time you feel distracted or feel that you just don't have what it takes to keep going, close your eyes for a moment and think of the people you just listed as your anchors. Imagine them saying, "You can do it." Or just silently say their names or mentally picture them smiling at you.

Mood words as anchors. Sports psychologists teach athletes to use "mood words" as self-suggestions to evoke desirable feelings when they play. For example, to feel strong, they might repeat to themselves words such as, "mighty," "muscles," "force," "power," or "strength." To feel confident, they might say, "bold," "great," "on-target," "in-control," or "terrific."

The best kind of mood word is onomatopoeia, a word that sounds like whatever it's describing. For example, in tennis, the sound of the word "pow" evokes feelings of power and accuracy—exactly what a player would hope for in a shot.

Check off the mood words that you think might help to you stay in a relaxed-alert state and add some of your own:

- ❏ *Calm*
- ❏ *Focused*
- ❏ *In my zone*
- ❏ *On-plan*
- ❏ *Can-do*
- ❏ _____
- ❏ _____

Here are some that sound a little like the mood itself. They lend themselves to steady repetition: for example, "Now, now, now, now, now."

- ❏ *Go*
- ❏ *Flow*
- ❏ *On*
- ❏ *Yes*
- ❏ *Now*
- ❏ _____
- ❏ _____

4. Affirmations

Every time you direct your attention onto your abilities, skills, and good qualities, you affirm them. And what you pay attention to will grow: attention is rewarding, and behavior that's rewarded gets repeated.

To compose an affirmation, think of the "three P's"—personal, positive, and present.

- *Personal*—Start with the pronoun "I."
- *Positive*—As with all self-talk, use "do," not "don't."
- *Present*—Choose a present-tense verb.

Here are some all-purpose examples. Choose your favorites and add your own:

- ❏ *I'm smart and I'm sharp.*
- ❏ *I'm getting this done today.*
- ❏ *I can do this.*
- ❏ *I have the focus-zone edge.*
- ❏ *I'm on it.*
- ❏ _____
- ❏ _____

5. Thought Substitution

We've already talked a lot about thought substitution. Let's practice with some examples of common distracting thoughts:

Unhelpful thought: I'll never get this done on time

Helpful counterthought: I'm good at what I do; if anyone can do it, I can.

Unhelpful thought: I just can't concentrate.

Helpful counterthought: I can concentrate. I've got lots of good tools to find my focus zone and stay there.

Unhelpful thought: I'm too tired to think. I'm on empty.

Helpful counterthought: I've got a reserve tank. Let's see what I can do. Then if I'm still too tired, I'll take a power break.

Here are some more unhelpful thoughts. It's your turn to come up with helpful counterthoughts:

Unhelpful perfectionist thought: I tried but I can't get it right.

Helpful counterthought: _____

_____

Unhelpful self-limiting thought: I can't learn this. I don't have what it takes.

Helpful counterthought: _____

_____

This time, jot down some of your own typical unhelpful thoughts. For each one, write out a counterthought that has enough oomph for you to substitute it successfully.

Unhelpful thought: _____

_____

Helpful counterthought: _____

_____

*Unhelpful thought:*_____

_____

Helpful counterthought: _____

_____

⚷ Attitude Shift

In the words of Winston Churchill, "Attitude is a little thing that makes a big difference." The way a pilot uses the word "attitude" reminds me of the direct link between attitude and results: A plane's attitude—the angle at which it flies—determines where it will go. If its attitude is looking up, you can climb to the sky. If it's level, you can go far. And if it's wrong when it's time to land, you crash.

In his book *Man's Search For Meaning*, psychologist and Holocaust survivor Viktor Frankl made this powerful observation:

> Everything can be taken from a man but one thing: the last of the human freedoms—to choose one's attitude in any given set of circumstances, to choose one's own way.

Don't Kill the Messenger

It's hard to have a good attitude about your clock when the alarm rings on Monday morning. Intellectually, the problem-solving part of your brain knows your clock is a useful tool. But the emotional part of your brain feels more like the old Roman generals who ordered bearers of bad news to be put to death. Smashing that clock seems like a satisfying option.

It's possible to hold both a positive and a negative view of something at the same time—to be ambivalent about it—and this is how we're prone to feel about clocks, calendars, schedule books, PDAs and to-do lists. We like them because they give us the structure that we want, but we hate them because they seem to be telling us what to do. Both "want to" and "have to" are in the mix.

It is part of the human condition that if we "have to," it's hard, but if we "want to," it's easy. So why do we make it so hard on ourselves and cling to the part of our ambivalence that says we "have to"? If we stop blaming the messengers and instead choose thoughts that help us like them better, we'll be more attracted to use our time management tools.

One helpful thought to keep in mind is that time is a measure of the length of life itself. In this light, clocks, calendars, schedule books, PDAs and to-do lists are our protective guardians. We all wish we had more time. That's exactly the reason we want to allocate time wisely and why these tools have such value to us.

Ticked Off by Your Clock?

Nick was sophomore at High Tech High, an innovative charter school in San Diego. Like most teenagers, Nick loved to stay up late at night on his computer or Game Cube. Nick was a video gamer and he had several favorites he'd become quite skilled at playing. Getting to bed at a decent time was a constant problem for Nick, and consequently so was getting up in the morning. Nick and his parents had tried multiple alarm clocks and behavior modification programs using reward charts and tokens. They had strict rules about the hours when Nick could play video games. But getting up on time remained a struggle. Nick wanted to do the right thing, but even when he got to bed on time, he'd lie awake thinking about his games and still oversleep in the morning.

Nick loved new technology. One day at a family counseling session, we discussed a new combination alarm clock and CD player that had just hit the market. You could set the alarm to play any track of music you chose. Nick and his parents made a pact that if he got the new alarm, he'd recommit to getting up. Nick agreed that if he didn't get up with it right away, the alarm would go back to the store. As an added incentive, Nick's parents agreed that for every morning Nick woke up with it, he could have ten bonus minutes of video games that night.

At home, Nick's younger sister came up with this idea: What

if they made a CD of the soundtrack of his favorite video game? Then when the alarm went off, Nick would instantly be connected with the promise of playing an extra ten minutes if he got up right away. Since game themes are intended to give you a jolt of adrenaline, it was an inspired idea. Nick downloaded the theme, which had a rapid, pulsating rhythm, and started to make peace with the tool he'd previously dreaded—his alarm clock.

Make Friends with Your Time Management Tools

Here are some tips for you to try:

- Give your PDA or schedule book a name that makes you smile, a distinctive case, or a wacky cover.
- Treat yourself to a clock or wristwatch that you really like.
- Get a daily tear-off calendar with a new joke every day.

Weed out your bad feelings about structure and schedules that may be left over from school days when you were forced to "color inside the lines." Replace them with pleasant associations that connect you with the valuable service these tools provide. As Christopher Robin says in A. A. Milne's *Winnie the Pooh*, "Organize is what you do before you do something. So that when you do it, it's not all mixed up."

Reframing

When you decide to see your time management tools as allies instead of enemies, you're using a powerful cognitive strategy called reframing. This practice of changing your point of view got its name because if you move the frame of a picture, you see the same thing but with a new focal point and perspective. Think of zooming in and out or moving side-to-side with a camera or a computer program like Mapquest. The level of detail and the center change as you choose new ways to frame your picture or map.

To stay on track, reframe your distracting thoughts. Give them new meaning by seeing them as useful signals telling you that you need to take action right away. If you keep losing your place when you read, make that your prompt to ask yourself if you need a power break. If it's a low-energy time of day, think, "I need a high-stim activity." When you start to get distracted, instead of passively letting your mind wander on and off, reframe your loss of focus as a cue for you to use a strategy to get back into your zone.

Reframing Failure and Mistakes

Winston Churchill also said, "Success is the ability to go from failure to failure without losing your enthusiasm." To do this, it helps to stay centered on your efforts and detached from any particular outcome. Life is a movie, not a still picture. If you define yourself by one particular win or loss, you'll get stuck in one frame while life moves on to the next.

If you make a decision that results in a loss, reframe it for what it is: a part of your ongoing efforts to learn and succeed. Instead of beating yourself up over it, say, *"Hey, I'm proud of myself for trying. What can I learn from that?"*

This is easier said than done. We all fill our heads with what we "should have done." We learned this at a very young age. In school we took tests that came back to us marked to show the answers we got wrong, not those we got right. Magazine ads show us airbrushed models with perfect faces and bodies that make us feel inferior when we look in the mirror. Listen in on any conversation about stock market investments. People are thrilled to tell you they bought Google stock at 89 but no one mentions having sold it at 100, before it went up to 500+. The cultural message is, "We expect you to be perfect, and if you're not, you're a loser. Feel bad about it." But the truth is that if you can't make a mistake, you can't make anything.

When you reframe making mistakes as having the guts to try, you are in good company. When he held the record, Babe Ruth hit more home runs than any other ball player, but he also struck out more times. The link is pretty obvious: he swung more times at the ball!

When you reframe making mistakes as feedback from which you can learn, you are rubbing elbows with genius. When asked about the results of his experiments to invent the lightbulb, Thomas

Edison's famous reply was: "Results! Why, man, I've gotten a lot of results. I know several thousand things that won't work."

The next time you make a mistake, reframe it as a step to success. In the words of basketball superstar Michael Jordan:

I've missed more than 9,000 shots in my career. I've lost almost 300 games. Twenty-six times I've been trusted to take a game-winning shot and missed. I've failed over and over and over again in my life. And that is why I succeed.

Reframing "Comfortable"

Think of the last time you visited a new city. On the day you arrived, everything seemed strange and unfamiliar. You probably felt kind of lost. But if you stayed there long enough, you found your way around. By the time you left, you knew where you were going and felt more comfortable there.

To be able to learn anything new, we need to tolerate an initial period of discomfort. This is sometimes called "coming out of your comfort zone." Your comfort zone is the circle of experience with which you are familiar. In your comfort zone, you feel content and relaxed. When you come outside your comfort zone, as you do when you're visiting a new city, you break out of your circle of experience. At first you may feel hyperalert and on your guard. But as you learn more about your new surroundings, you feel more at ease. Your comfort zone expands into a larger circle.

Your comfort zone is *not* the same as your focus zone. *In fact, sometimes you need to leave your comfort zone to find your focus zone.* If you're too comfortable, you'll get bored and be too understimulated to focus. You have to venture outside your comfort zone to get the novelty and adrenaline you need to feel alert and alive.

In counseling, when I introduce people to a psychological tool for the first time—rescripting the past or mental rehearsal, for instance—many will hesitate or decline at first. They'll say, "This doesn't feel comfortable to me." Then, a week later, they recognize that "not feeling comfortable" was actually their resistance to change. They decide to overcome their resistance and tolerate some temporary discomfort. And when they see results, they're glad they did.

If you feel uncomfortable about trying cognitive strategies, listen with new ears to what you're saying to yourself. Reframe your discomfort as a sign that you're learning new skills.

The next time you need to reframe feeling comfortable, what self-talk will you use?

- ❑ *Good. This means I'm learning.*
- ❑ *I'm glad it feels so different. If I were doing all the same things, why would I expect different results?*
- ❑ *I want to feel alive! I want adventure and discovery!*

Reframing Fear of Missing Out (FOMO)

When my daughters were in high school, the three of us were invited to appear on a TV talk show, *State of Mind*, cablecast by the University of California at San Diego (UCSD). On one segment of the show, my daughters were part of a roundtable discussion with other teens. Not surprisingly, the topic of overcommitting to activities came up. One young man said he felt defeated because he had to give up playing on a baseball team that spring. The other kids all commiserated.

I knew that my daughters were struggling with this same issue themselves. I listened carefully as they encouraged him to look at it a different way. "You know you're not defeated because you can't play ball this year," my older daughter wisely said. "You're a winner because you're prioritizing. It's what good decision makers do."

The boy was noticeably happier. (I'm sure it helped that an attractive teenage girl delivered this advice.) He reframed having to say no, and saw it instead as saying yes—to being a capable leader of his own life.

Reframing is a powerful antidote to FOMO—the fear of missing out, which you read about in Chapter 6. Instead of feeling as if others have an edge on you because they're doing something you cannot do, you turn it around so that you feel *you* have the edge because you're mature, decisive, and in control.

Next time you need to say no but it's hard, reframe it as a plus, not a minus. Practice helpful self-talk so you are prepared:

❑ *I'm proud of myself for prioritizing.*

❑ *I'm glad I have the backbone to be a good decision maker.*

❑ *If I just keep saying yes, then I am missing out—on being in charge of my own life.*

⚷ Mental Rehearsal

In Chapter 6, you read about one instance of mental rehearsal when Mary prepared to retake the bar exam. Mental rehearsal is a visualization technique. When visualization is used along with adequate preparation and work, it can help to improve results. Mary repeatedly pictured taking the bar exam in her focus zone, and this helped her break the self-defeating pattern of what had happened to her the last time.

The Swedish sports psychologist Dr. Lars-Eric Unestahl made another valuable contribution to the field when he observed something interesting about top athletes as they mentally rehearsed: not only did they practice their physical form, but they also rehearsed exactly how they wanted to feel. It is now widely recognized that mental rehearsal can help you control both your emotions and your focus when you perform, especially when you need to stay cool under pressure.

Athletes use mental rehearsal for weeks before an important competition. They continue to practice what they want to think, feel, and do, right up to the moment they actually think, feel, and do it. When they're visualizing before an event, they call it a "precompetition strategy." When they're visualizing during an event, that's called a "competition strategy."

You can do the same thing for yourself, when it's important for you to stay in your focus zone. If you have a major event, such as a big exam, board meeting, or speaking engagement, you can mentally rehearse how you want to feel, as well as what you want to think and do. When you practice it ahead of time, it's your "pre-concentration strategy." Then when you're there, and you want to recapture what you have practiced, visualize how you want to feel right there on the spot. This is your "concentration strategy."

Relax When You Mentally Rehearse

Visualization works best when you're in a relaxed, receptive state. Many athletes use progressive muscle relaxation exercises before they mentally rehearse. They tense and relax each muscle group, as you learned to do as a change-of-state key in Chapter 5. Some athletes prefer self-hypnosis to feel relaxed and receptive, and others like to meditate. Before you start to mentally rehearse, decide how you will relax—muscle relaxation, four-corner breathing, relaxing imagery. Choose whatever method works best for you.

Use Anchors for Mental Rehearsal

When you mentally rehearse, it's helpful to use a keyword or symbol to connect yourself back to your rehearsal. For example, if you're practicing how you want to feel during an important sales presentation, you might repeat the word "confident" as you rehearse. Then, on that day, when you say the word "confident," you'll connect back to the confidence you felt when you rehearsed.

Write a Letter to Your Future Self

When you anticipate a challenge in your future, send reinforcements ahead. Choose a time when you feel strong and resolved. Then write a note to yourself that you can read later on, when you need the strength and determination you feel now.

Ginny was on a weight management program, but sometimes after a hectic day at the office, when she came home, she compulsively overate. While she was still feeling resolute, she wrote herself this note. She left it on the hall table to read after she came through the front door—but before she hit the kitchen—in case it had been a particularly stressful day at work:

Dear Ginny,

Slow down. Take some deep breaths. Think of all your hard work cooking balanced meals and going to spinning classes at the gym. Keep the drive alive! Stay focused on how you want to look and feel in your new jeans. You can do it. I believe in you.

Ginny

This technique is particularly useful for parents who want to stop being homework police. When you're talking with your child and he's in a cooperative mood, explain that you'd like to stop having to tell him when it's time to do homework. It feels like nagging and neither of you likes that. Ask him to write a note to his future self. It can be simple, funny, text-message slang—whatever works.

Hey Dude,

Sit down & start working. Get it done so U can go outside & play.

This is ME talking 2 U.

Let him keep the original, and you keep a copy. The next time he's dawdling when it's time to start his homework, give him a chance to remember to find his own note and read it. If he doesn't, quietly hand him your copy. That way, you're out of the loop. He's telling himself that's it time to begin.

Looking Ahead

Does your lifestyle help or hurt your ability to pay attention? In Chapter 9, you'll learn behavior skills—healthy habits—to keep you living in your focus zone.

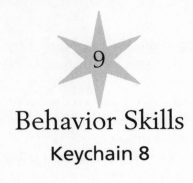

Behavior Skills
Keychain 8

A man walks into a doctor's office with a banana in one ear, a cucumber in the other, and a pickle up his nose. He asks, "Hey, doc, what's wrong with me?" The doctor looks at him and replies, "You're not eating right."

—OLD VAUDEVILLE JOKE

Behavior skills are the actions we choose every day that turn into the habits that make us who we are. The right daily habits can increase your basic ability to stay in your focus zone. In this chapter, you'll learn the eighth and last keychain, a new set of keys to keep your brain fit and focused:

Keychain 8 ⚷ Healthy Habits

Be patient with yourself when you decide to make a lifestyle change. New habits take time, persistence, lots of self-encouragement, and instant self-forgiveness. It helps to keep in mind that the brain is adaptable and changes with your new choices, as you read about in Chapter 4. The more you practice, the more you strengthen your new brain pathways, so maintaining your new habits gets easier with time.

The healthy-habits keychain includes three sturdy keys: lifestyles of the calm and focused; supportive friends; and living clutter-free.

Self-defeating habits are hard to break. Regardless of whether your actions help or hurt you, it's a natural human tendency to justify them to yourself, so you can avoid cognitive dissonance. Essentially, "cognitive dissonance" means that you cannot hold two conflicting thoughts at the same time. So, for instance, if you believe in efficiency and then you procrastinate, your brain instantly assumes that there's a reason for the procrastination. And that reason, or a variation of it, will justify your procrastination again tomorrow.

To prevent getting caught by cognitive dissonance, you need objectivity—your observer self. You need to put some emotional distance between you and your actions so you can see what you're doing and challenge your justifications. A detached, big-picture perspective lets you accept your need to improve in a self-aware, matter-of-fact way.

Imagine yourself in a small plane at an altitude of about 3,000 feet (914 meters). Houses, people, and cars look like miniatures in a model train set. From the plane, you can look down to earth and see yourself and your current habits. Now stay at 3,000 feet as you read this chapter. Your bird's-eye view will help you make lifestyle choices that favor attention control.

Keychain 8 ⊶ Healthy Habits

- Lifestyles of the Calm and Focused
- Supportive Friends
- Living Clutter-Free

⊶ Lifestyles of the Calm and Focused

We're all well aware of what it means to have a healthy lifestyle, but most of us have room for improvement. It helps to know the rationale for recommendations you're trying to follow, and to understand the impact of your choices on your ability to focus. In this section, we'll cover: (1) sufficient sleep; (2) good nutrition; (3) the savvy use of stimulants; (4) physical fitness; and (5) fun and relaxation.

1. Sufficient Sleep

What time did you go to bed last night? What time did you wake up this morning? Did you sleep through the night without waking up? How many hours? Is this your usual routine?

Although individual needs vary, most adults do best with about eight hours of sleep. Research suggests that signs of sleep deprivation—including a diminished capacity for focused attention—usually start to occur in adults with less than seven hours of sleep. If you sleep seven hours or less, you need more sleep—and you're not alone. More than 60 percent of Americans sleep less than seven hours per night.

Current research shows a strong link between lack of sleep and attention deficit disorder (ADD). People who are sleep-deprived show symptoms that mimic ADD, and approximately 70 to 80 percent of all people with ADD have difficulty sleeping. The most common problem is slowing the brain down to get to sleep.

Another common sleep problem is a catch-22 with caffeine. If you didn't sleep last night, you'll use more caffeine today, which will make you lose sleep again tonight.

Tips for getting better sleep include:

- Reduce your caffeine, and only drink it early in the day.
- Go to bed and wake up at about the same time each day.
- No high-stim activity before bedtime, especially TV violence or horror.
- Practice relaxing bedtime rituals, such as pleasant music and inspirational reading.
- Make your bedroom a stress-free sanctuary, with no reminders of work or things you have to do.

2. Good Nutrition

Balanced brain chemistry begins with balanced eating. Food is the raw material from which brain chemicals are built. To have the stamina to go the distance when you've got to focus, you need fuel that burns slowly and lasts.

Sugar. Current research on attention deficit disorder suggests that for most children with this diagnosis, sugar doesn't cause their ADD symptoms. The National Institutes of Health conducted double-blind studies in which parents, staff members, and children did not know which days children with ADD had sugar or not. No noticeable differences in behavior and learning were reported between sugar and no-sugar days. Other studies show that the "Feingold diet," which eliminates food additives and refined sugar, results in decreased symptoms for only about 5 percent of children with ADD.

These research findings are informative, but they don't replace common sense. From whenever the tradition of giving birthday parties for small children began, mothers have known to serve the cake and ice cream last. The brain metabolizes glucose, a form of sugar that the body makes from the foods you eat. Complex carbohydrates convert to glucose slowly; refined sugar converts almost instantly. In this way, your energy patterns correspond to the blood-sugar level in your body.

At any age—and whether or not you have ADD—you can get a rush from too much sugar, but later you'll get burned out. It's best to use sugar wisely and stay on an even keel.

The blood-brain barrier. Both alcohol and caffeine affect focused attention. To make good decisions about them, it helps to understand the blood-brain barrier. Composed of nearly 400 miles of highly specialized capillaries, this boundary protects our brains at a microscopic level. It keeps out almost all the chemicals that pass freely through the rest of the body, but allows water and essential nutrients to pass through. Because of their simple molecular structure, some drugs such as alcohol, nicotine, and caffeine get in, too. That's why they produce changes in how you think and feel. They've made it past the barrier to act directly on the brain.

The blood-brain barrier is like a tough secretary who controls access to the boss's office. It allows the brain to carry on vital functions and not waste precious energy on needless or damaging interruptions. So if you want to decrease your consumption of alcohol or caffeine, instead of seeing yourself as having to give up your evening wine or afternoon Red Bull, you can reframe your choice another way. In real life, we all know that the more important the CEO, the harder it is to get through the door. So imagine that you now have an even tougher new secretary, because your prefrontal CEO—the part of your brain that keeps you in your focus zone—is just that important.

Alcohol. In moderation, alcohol is relaxing and fun. It's good for recreation, but not for mental acuity. It starts to blur your thinking after just one drink. It slows reflexes, weakens short-term memory, and induces loss of inhibition, which makes it hard to resist distraction. Different people metabolize alcohol at different rates, but most people achieve a blood alcohol concentration of .02 to .03 percent with each drink, and process it at the rate of .01 to .015 percent per hour.

As a point of reference, in most states you are "likely DUI" (driving under the influence) between .05 and .07 percent, and "definitely DUI" at .08 percent. Weakened attention is noticeable at as low as .02 percent, and normal attention is not restored right away. That's because alcohol increases the turnover of dopamine and norepinephrine. So after you drink, you need recovery time to replenish these brain chemicals, which are critical for staying in your focus zone.

If you become too intoxicated, you may not resume functioning at your best level of focus for a day or two. That's because alcohol disrupts the "architecture" of your sleep. In other words, it breaks the cycle of brain waves that leads to a state of REM (rapid eye movement) or dream sleep, which you need to replenish your brain chemicals. In sleep labs when subjects are allowed to sleep but not allowed to enter a state of REM, they remain sleep-deprived and depleted. For the same reason, when you have jet lag, which you'll read about in Chapter 11, it takes longer to recover if you drink alcohol.

Caffeine. Worldwide, the only beverage consumed more than tea is water—although coffee may be catching up. According to an article in *National Geographic* (January 2005), "Every working day, Starbucks opens four new outlets somewhere on the planet and hires 200 new employees."

Caffeine stimulates the central nervous system. In moderation it increases alertness, reduces fatigue, and improves performance on mental tasks that require sustained attention, especially in monotonous conditions. When you use too much caffeine, the side effects include nervousness, jitteriness, and anxiety. Although it prolongs wakefulness, caffeine does *not* replace the need for sleep. When the effects wear off, what went up must come down.

Caffeine is rapidly absorbed into the bloodstream. Its average half-life—the time required by the body to eliminate one-half of the amount consumed—is three to seven hours. In other words, at seven o'clock in the evening you're still metabolizing about half of the caffeine from the latte you drank at two in the afternoon; and at eleven that night you're still running on one-fourth of it. It takes about fifteen to thirty-five hours to eliminate 95 percent of it.

Caffeine's half-life is hugely variable. It depends on age and a broad range of other factors. Smoking cuts it in half, and taking birth control pills doubles it. This is useful to keep in mind if everyone else orders coffee while you're trying to cut back. Don't compare yourself with others. Your brain and your situation are individual to you.

It helps to know the approximate caffeine content of what you're eating or drinking. *National Geographic* and a report from Stanford University list these amounts:

Coffee, brewed, 12 oz ("tall" in Starbucks)—200 mg
Coffee, instant, 12 oz (forbidden in Starbucks)—145 mg
Coffee, decaffeinated, 12 oz—7.6 mg
Espresso, 6 oz—240 mg
Tea, black, 8 oz—50 mg
Tea, green, 8 oz—30 mg
Soft drink, cola, 20 oz—57 mg

Soft drink, Mountain Dew, 64 oz (Double Big Gulp)—294 mg
Energy drink, Red Bull, 8.3 oz—80 mg
Excedrin pain reliever, 2 tablets—130 mg
Chocolate, 6 oz—25 mg

3. The Savvy Use of Stimulants

Now that you understand what it takes to stay in your focus zone, you can see the benefit of using stimulants strategically. They can boost your activation level by producing more adrenaline in your brain. But, as you read in Chapter 3, the more you use them, the more you build a tolerance for them. The same amount no longer gives you the same level of boost, so you're drawn to use more to keep getting the same response.

Stimulants are attractive; but as a habit, it's best to use them at low enough levels so that when you need to tackle a boring job or unusually long hours, you don't have to go to extremes. Low levels will keep you alert. In a monthlong study at Brigham and Women's Hospital in Boston, sixteen subjects took a pill every waking hour, without knowing if it was a placebo or caffeine. Results showed that frequent small amounts of daytime caffeine maintained alertness better than a large morning dose comparable to a big cup of coffee when you first wake up.

To use a stimulant wisely, consider how much you need, how long you'll need it, and how close to bedtime you are.

Caffeine as a strategy. Often we drink more caffeine than we need—not just because we've built a tolerance for it, but because that's the way it comes on the menu. It's not good marketing to call a product "small."

At Starbucks, you can order Tall, Grande, and Venti. (Some locations have a short cup available, but none list it on the menu board.) When your purpose is to break up your boredom, you'll be drawn to order the largest size so you can sip it as long as possible. But you can sip a decaf Venti for the same amount of time that you can sip a caffeinated one. And you can fine-tune how much caffeine you consume by requesting a specific blend of both. Let's take a look at the math. (These estimates are for coffees such as house blends and the coffee of the week, not espresso or specialty beverages.)

Size	Decaffeinated	Caffeinated	Decaf/Caf Blend
Tall (12 oz)	7.6 mg	200 mg	7.6 to 200 mg
Grande (16 oz)	10 mg	267 mg	10 to 267 mg
Venti (20 oz)	12.5 mg	334 mg	12.5 to 334 mg

When you ask for half caf and half decaf, or two-thirds decaf and one-third caf, you give yourself more choices and more control. In fact, "fading" is a useful method for periodically cutting down on your caffeine. Over time, you gradually decrease the caffeinated coffee and increase the decaffeinated coffee in the blend that you order or brew at home. Some people prefer to go cold turkey every so often, to recalibrate their caffeine intake at a lower dose (and their spouses prefer to go out of town when they do).

Electronic stimulation. The rise of electronic entertainment today is unprecedented. On one hand, high-quality programs provide informative news, complex narratives, and hip humor. Many video games improve logic, abstract reasoning, and coordination—skills that carry over to other areas of life. In one study, for instance, surgeons who played Super Monkey Ball for more than three hours per week had better skills in laparoscopic surgery—a procedure that uses a tiny camera and joystick-controlled tools to cut and suture—than those who did not.

On the other hand, television can waste time, numb your mind, and weaken family bonds. An alarming 66 percent of Americans regularly watch TV while eating dinner instead of talking to each other and reconnecting after a day at work or school. Most addiction centers now offer treatment for abuse of the Internet and video games such as EverQuest, which has also been dubbed "EverCrack." We are forging new ground in the use of electronic stimulation, discovering its rewards and its risks.

Flicker. We do not yet know the effects on our brains of electronic flicker, the pulses of light that fire rapidly from the video screen to the brain. The knowledge that a flickering light can cause alterations in consciousness is as old as the discovery of fire. Ancient shamans and bards used the magic of campfires to enhance the power of their storytelling.

Scientists developed an instrument called the tachistoscope to study the effects of flicker. They found that it alters brain wave patterns, but that not all flicker is alike. The flame of a campfire induces a relaxing EEG pattern known as brain coherence; but the flicker from television and video, while still having a hypnotic attraction, has disruptive effects on brain waves.

Television and attention. A study published in the medical journal *Pediatrics* shows a strong connection between TV watching at early ages and weak attention later on. Researchers related the hours of television watched by 1,300 children ages one to three with their scores on measures of attention problems at age seven. Frequent viewers were most likely to score in the highest 10 percent for having problems concentrating. Every added hour of watching TV increased a child's risk of having problems by 10 percent. The American Academy of Pediatrics now recommends *no* television for children from birth to two years of age.

Electronics and self-awareness. To stay balanced when you're plugged into your electronics, practice the self-awareness keys you learned in Chapter 5. Get in the habit of asking yourself, "What am I *not* doing now?" Unlike reading a book, you'll never get to the last page of the Internet, so you have to decide when to quit and go spend time with your family, friends, or nature. In Chapter 10, you'll learn more tips to stay productive when you're browsing or searching the Internet.

Freedom from stimulant abuse. Any time you use a drug, you get the good with the bad, the benefits with the risks and costs. Some stimulants are a bad trade. They pump your adrenaline and increase your alertness, but hurt your brain and your body. You pay way too much for the good that you get.

In today's world, stimulants have a strong pull on us, and we each have different thresholds for addiction. If you think you may need professional treatment, go for it. Think of how good it'll feel to get your life back in balance.

4. Physical Fitness

Regular exercise lowers the levels of your stress chemicals. With less norepinephrine, your brain keeps a balanced chemistry so you can stay in your focus zone.

In my practice, I've seen marked improvement in people's capacity to stay calm and focused once they've adopted an exercise routine. As one woman put it, "After I exercise, my head is on straight."

Some sports, such as the martial arts, tennis, and golf, require that you learn and continually practice focus skills. But any activity that gets you moving will help you replenish the brain chemicals you need for mental clarity and decrease the ones that make you distraction-prone.

What's the best sport to keep you in your focus zone? The answer is simple. It's the sport that *you* like enough to get out there and play.

5. Relaxation and Fun

Meditation, biofeedback, self-hypnosis, yoga, practicing your faith, having peaceful family dinners . . . Any routine activity that decreases tension also improves your attention.

Brain imaging studies suggest that daily meditators derive particular benefit, as you read in Chapter 4. In my practice, I've worked with people who enjoy meditation, and I've worked with people who try it but find it isn't right for them. Meditation is a time-honored and powerful practice to improve daily focus. However, you need to find what works for you. Start with something simple that you enjoy, like going for a walk.

In Chapter 5, you learned relaxation methods to reduce your adrenaline score when you're tense, provoked, or caught in a state of fight-or-flight. If you'd like to see real improvement in your overall capacity to stay calm under pressure, try taking some time *every day* to relax.

Relaxation and avoidance. Sometimes it's hard to relax, because thoughts and feelings you'd rather not deal with can surface. In fact, many people keep themselves overly busy mainly to avoid unpleasant emotions such as guilt, resentment, or anxiety.

Doing something else is a good coping mechanism when you can't do anything about the source of your problems, as you read in Chapter 6 when you learned about thought substitution. But if staying busy is your automatic answer to feeling bad, you thwart your ability to solve your problems.

When you slow down to relax, if you find you feel sad, agitated, or anxious, see what happens when you take the time to ask yourself why. Are you lonely? Mad at someone? Nervous about money? Then see what happens when you address your problem calmly and look for a rational solution.

Gary, a busy, ambitious real estate agent, usually made time for his family even with his full schedule. Recently, however, he was staying late at the office, taking work home, and holding long open houses on Sundays. His wife finally insisted on a relaxing weekend together. At first Gary protested, but his wife made arrangements for them to stay overnight at his favorite mountain lodge. Driving home on Sunday, they talked about good times they'd shared together. As they reminisced, Gary thought about his coming birthday, and for the first time he connected his recent frenzied behavior with the fact that he was about to turn forty. He confided in his wife that he had hoped to be an independent broker by this point in his life. The tension left his body as he acknowledged this, and they began the first of many conversations to make a plan for Gary to start his own business.

Avoidance is like having a leaky roof. When it rains, it's too wet to go up on the roof to fix the leak; but when it's sunny, who cares about a leaky roof? When you're in crisis mode or doing damage control after a storm has occurred in your life, you don't have the time or psychological resources to figure out how to stop getting hurt from such storms. But when a storm is over, you can—unless you bury yourself in distraction by staying busy.

Hard-driving type A personalities say that they cannot relax. If this describes you, practice the strategy of reframing. Decide that you will tolerate the initial discomfort of learning to do something new. Then watch as this simple new habit gives you added power to stay focused and balanced.

Learning to relax. Buddhist monks who meditate daily can lower their heart rate and control other supposedly involuntary functions of the autonomic nervous system that most people can't control consciously. You can raise your right arm, for instance, instantly and directly. But if you want to lower your heart rate, you need to be still and invite relaxation using a more subtle method called "passive volition."

One method to decrease the functioning of the autonomic system that has been shown to be effective is the "relaxation response," developed by Herbert Benson, MD. This method consists of four steps:

1. Close your eyes.
2. Relax your muscles.
3. Breathe slowly and deeply.
4. Repeat a simple, calming word or phrase to yourself. Benson suggests the word "one."

A visit from aliens. When I teach passive volition in stress management workshops, I use this story to describe how it works:

Let's say an alien has landed on earth, and he comes from a planet where there is no such thing as sleep. He sees us sleeping, and we look so peaceful. And he hears us talk about outrageous fantasies we call dreams. He wants to learn how to sleep, too. What would you tell him?

People usually give answers like, "Find a dark, quiet place," "Lie down and close your eyes," and "Count sheep."

I reply, "Exactly. Put all these answers together and what you're telling him is to imitate a sleeping person until he becomes one. And that's the best definition of passive volition that I know. *You imitate a relaxed person until you become one.*"

Appreciation. In the 1970s, I had the privilege of participating in one of the last teaching conferences conducted by Hans Selye, MD, the discoverer of biological stress. Dr. Selye taught us that the only thoughts strong enough to compete with stress are thoughts of appreciation. I tucked that idea away because it resonated with what was true for me. When I felt bombarded by the demands of graduate school—papers due, exams, having more month left than money—I could feel better by repeating statements of gratitude: *"I'm thankful to have this opportunity." "I'm grateful for all that I'm learning." "I'm glad for the money I do have."*

Years later, as scientists learned more about brain chemicals, it became clear that Dr. Selye truly was ahead of his time. It turns out that when we feel gratitude we promote serotonin, which slows down the cascade of stress chemicals. In other words, thoughts of gratitude decrease the fight-or-flight brain chemical, norepinephrine, and return us to a relaxed-alert state.

You may have already discovered this effect for yourself. Next time you're under fire from the demands that surround you, remember to use appreciative self-talk to defeat your stress:

- *I'm thankful for my life, health, family, friends, and home.*
- *I'm grateful for today.*
- *I'm glad for all that I have.*
- *I'm especially thankful for _____.*
- *At this moment, I feel grateful for _____.*

Humor. Fun is a natural stimulant, and laughter reduces tension. We tend to think that to increase our focus, we have to get more serious. The opposite is usually true. To sustain focus, we usually need to lighten up.

There is an old joke about three passengers on a small plane: an old priest, a college kid, and the smartest man in the world. The engine quits and the pilot bails out, but before he jumps, he tells them that there are only two parachutes left. The smartest man in the world pronounces that he has a responsibility to posterity to save himself, and before anyone can protest, he is gone, too. The elderly priest turns to the student and says, "Take the last parachute, my son. I've had a long and full life, and yours has just begun." "No worries, Father," says the boy. "The smartest man in the world just jumped out of this plane with my knapsack."

Faith, not fear. When you believe in yourself—your abilities, your future, and the possibilities in your life—you build a strong brain chemistry that sustains your focus and motivation. It helps to use encouraging self-talk, such as "*I can learn this*"; or to repeat anchor words, such as "*trust*" or "*yes.*"

Athletes say, "*I can do this*," when they're stretching their limits, trying to run another mile farther or bench-press ten more pounds. When you feel you can't face a boring but necessary task because it's too dull or you're too distracted, give it a try. Say, "*I can do this*" sincerely, the way you'd support a good friend.

In a sense, the mythic battle between faith and fear is fought on the molecular level. Persistent self-statements of faith and confidence increase serotonin, regulate dopamine, and keep norepinephrine in check. Faith wins; fear loses. But when you let fear and self-doubt take over, norepinephrine dominates. Fear wins; faith loses.

Use every cognitive strategy you can think of—self-talk, reframing, thought substitution—to keep your faith in yourself. When you do, you generate brain chemicals that help you sustain your focus.

⌐ Supportive Friends

If you want to promote focus in your life, choose friends who value it, too. Mirror neurons—the brain's mechanism for social learning—cause us to influence and be influenced by our companions. If your friends have structure and balance in their lives, you will naturally mirror those qualities.

A friend can help you achieve your goals or unintentionally help you move farther away from them. If your friends have meaningful goals, you'll support each other's efforts to stay focused. If they lack goals or are obsessed by goals, they're likely to pull you with them to one side of the inverted U or the other.

Everyone needs to vent, but friends who complain a lot drain your energy. Set a ten-minute limit on venting. For better or worse, our brains tend to synchronize with the brains of those with whom we spend time. So make mirror neurons work in your favor.

A Mentor Can Be a Friend

In times of stress, it's especially important to have friends who support you. That friend can be a peer, a family member, or even a mentor.

When I was doing my internship at Parkland Memorial Hospital in Dallas, Texas, I was there on a rotation with a brilliant young resident who was on an international fellowship. Far from his own home and family, he was starting to break under the heavy demands of the program. He was showing up late for rounds, lagging behind in his paperwork, and losing his ability to concentrate. The year was 1975, before the age of modern antidepressants. I felt helpless, as did the other interns in the program. We were barely keeping up ourselves and could not take on his load too.

The chief of psychiatry took this young man under his wing. They talked and agreed that, for the time being, the chief would personally give him a wake-up phone call every day, and three times a week they'd go for a run. The difference this simple practice made was astonishing. In a matter of weeks, the intern resumed his usual high level of performance.

Buddies Make a Difference

If you have a goal or project for which you need a motivational boost, call a friend with a similar interest and set up a date to meet. Research shows that the buddy system increases follow-through for people trying to stick with new routines, such as physical exercise. Also, if you work at home, having even one appointment in your book adds structure to your day.

Think of three friends who support you. How do your nurture these friendships? When is the last time *you* called? Initiating a contact sends the message that you're thinking about the other person.

Write the names of these three supportive people, the last time you contacted them, and when you plan to be in contact again:

Supportive Friend	Last Contact	Next Contact

The best way to have a supportive friend is to be one. Take time to support your friends:

- Contact them on a regular basis. Put it in your schedule book or PDA.
- Let them know you value the friendship.
- Be a good listener. Be willing to give them your undivided attention.

When I think about mirror neurons, I'm reminded that we're all hardwired to be social creatures. I have the same thought when I watch children at play. Sometimes all they want is to spend time with a good friend. It makes them feel happier and stronger.

Robert Louis Stevenson once said, "A friend is a gift you give yourself." Be the best gift your friend can get, and give yourself the very best, too.

⚫⚖ Living Clutter-Free

Clutter is distracting. Your eyes and your brain have too many places to wander. Photos, artwork, and pleasing decorations provide stimulation that helps you stay in your focus zone. But piles of paper and stacks of stuff are petty thieves that sap you of your attention.

Clutter is deferred decision making. Think about it for a moment. What's the real reason you don't want to deal with that file, magazine article, financial record, old letter, or child's artwork? It's indecision, isn't it? You don't want to throw it away, but you don't want to commit to keeping it, either. So into a stack it goes.

It's no problem to throw away junk mail. And it's no problem keeping records you'll need for your tax returns. But what do you do with all that stuff in between? You don't know for sure. And because uncertainty causes anxiety, you duck the decision by putting it off. "For now" you can put it on that shelf over there.

We all know: Handle paperwork only once. Act on it, then file it or toss it. But this is like saying, "Eat your vegetables." *The problem isn't knowing what to do; it's doing what we know*. This is true of clearing all kinds of clutter—computer files, household items, even social obligations. One way to improve is to understand the psychological forces behind clutter and then outsmart them.

Loss Aversion

In 2002, Daniel Kahneman, PhD, shared the Nobel Prize in economics for his work on human decision making under conditions of uncertainty. He and Amos Tversky, PhD, conducted a series of experiments that showed how emotions affect decisions, and how framing affects emotions.

Their findings showed that human beings demonstrate loss aversion. In other words, people will risk more to avoid a loss than to realize a gain. In one study, when given a hypothetical choice between getting $3,000 with certainty or having an 80/20 chance of getting $4,000, about 80 percent of all respondents chose the sure $3,000. But when given the same choice to lose $3,000 with certainty or take the same 80/20 chance on losing $4,000, only 8 percent opted for the sure $3,000 loss. Most people—in this case, 92 percent—didn't want to face the moment when they'd have to part with something of value, so they put it off and hoped they wouldn't have to do it at all.

Loss aversion helps explain the accumulation of clutter. We aren't certain what's of value and what's not. So we put the decision off, even if we wind up losing more. We'll give up our living space rather than come face-to-face with the pang of throwing something away that we might need later.

The Endowment Effect

Another force contributing to clutter is the endowment effect: Most people who are given an object will instantly value it more than they did before they received it and more than others value it.

The best-known demonstration of this effect is an experiment conducted at Cornell University, in which researchers randomly gave students either a mug or a chocolate bar, with identical market values. Beforehand, the researchers had established that half of the students preferred each item. Afterwards, they gave all the participants a chance to trade. Only 10 percent made the swap, compared to the 50 percent that would have been predicted strictly by economics theory.

The contents of your house have more value to you than they do to anyone else—you chose them; you use them; they meet your individual needs. According to the endowment effect, though, you value them for reasons beyond the functions that they serve. You value them for the simple reason that they are yours.

Fight Back by Reframing

Research on decision making shows that the way you phrase a question can change the outcome you get. In one survey, people were willing to accept inflation to reduce unemployment from 10 percent to 5 percent, but not to increase employment from 90 to 95 percent. *Our actions often depend on the way choices are presented.*

To clear clutter, reframe the questions you ask yourself when you're about to defer your decision. Think less about what you might lose if you delete something, and more about what you certainly will gain: space, order, and an efficient workspace.

Here's some reassuring self-talk to get past the pangs of loss. Add your own, too:

- ❏ *I'm creating space—to work, to relax, to breathe.*
- ❏ *When my desk is clear, my thinking is, too.*
- ❏ *I feel more relaxed when I can see open space in front of me.*
- ❏ *An orderly room, an orderly mind.*
- ❏ *I'll save time looking for things.*
- ❏ *I like the feeling of knowing I can find what I need when I need it.*
- ❏ *I like feeling free. I own my things; they do not own me.*

- ❏ _____

- ❏ _____

Another way to thwart loss aversion is to reframe the concept of loss itself, and give it a positive connotation. For example, you can use the metaphor of weight loss, which most of us regard as desirable. Try these and add your own:

- ❏ *I like to feel lean—in my body, my office, and my house.*
- ❏ *It takes months for me to shed extra pounds, but I can lose this weight in one afternoon.*
- ❏ *In my workspace, less is more.*

- ❏ _____

For Sentimental Reasons

In some ways, it's harder to eliminate clutter at home, because of the personal memories we attach to our things. How can we part with stuffed animals, old greeting cards, and souvenirs when they connect us with feelings we want to keep all our lives?

On one hand, digital technology is an enormous help. You can take photos of keepsakes before you let them go. This is especially helpful for children when they have to say good-bye to favorite toys that they've outgrown. On the other hand, digital technology is responsible for new forms of clutter. When cameras used film, you'd have about ten photos of a special event. Now, by the time others send you their digital photos of the event too, you have hundreds. As computer sizes grow in gigabytes, digital clutter does too.

You can reduce digital clutter by sitting down, organizing your files, making the best use of your software, and adding an external drive. Chapter 10 will give you more ideas for getting organized at your computer. But giving up old books, tapes, and knickknacks requires a harder kind of emotional letting go. You need to say good-bye to the experience of holding those memories in your hands.

A useful reframing for clearing clutter at home is to make yourself look forward, not backward, in time. The space you create is your living space for the future. When you give your discards to charity, they'll do more good for someone else than they're doing for you now. Think more about where you're going and less about where you've been.

Here's some helpful self-talk for letting go of home clutter:

- ❏ *These memories are in my heart, where they matter most.*
- ❏ *I trust in life to give me what I need to recall these feelings anytime I want.*
- ❏ *Someone else could use this much more than I can.*
- ❏ *I'm grateful I had this, and I look forward to what comes next.*

(And right now, that's Part III.)

Part III

Digital-Age Strategies for Success

With new keys jingling in your pocket, you'll want to put them to good use right away. Some will unlock answers to the daily problems that you face, and some are ignition keys to give you the drive and focus to achieve your personal goals.

In Part III you'll learn how to use your new keys in today's world of distraction. Chapter 10 explains how they can help you to manage interruptions and overload. Chapter 11 shows you ways to use them if you work from home or on the road. And Chapter 12 gives you new ways to understand attention deficit disorder (ADD) and how you'll benefit from using your keys if you have ADD or if your child has it.

By putting the eight keychains into practice, *everyone can defeat distraction and overload.*

10

Outsmarting Interruption
and Overload

*You are receiving this automatic notification because I am
out of the office. If I was in, chances are you wouldn't have
received any reply at all.*

—#1 ON LIST OF "BEST OUT-OF-OFFICE AUTO
REPLIES" CIRCULATED ON THE INTERNET, 2006

This chapter covers strategies for two ever-present workplace problems in today's world of distraction: interruptions and overload. In fact, if you started to read this chapter at work, you've probably already been interrupted by now.

Handling Interruptions

Gloria Mark, PhD, is a professor of informatics. In 2004, after shadowing office workers in high-tech firms for over 1,000 hours, she and her research team at the University of California, Irvine, reported that employees spent an average of eleven minutes working on a project before they were interrupted and had to shift to another task. It then took an average of twenty-five minutes to get back to their original task.

Dr. Mark's study showed something else: not all interruptions are bad. Often the call or e-mail that disrupted a worker's concentration brought exactly the information that the worker needed. This finding agreed with earlier research published in the *Academy of Management Review*. Interruptions are intrinsic to the way we work today; some experts say that we are "interrupt-driven." It's senseless to talk about eliminating interruptions. Our real goal is to improve the way we handle them.

Your Focus Zone in Outer Space

Writing for the *New York Times* (October 16, 2005), Clive Thompson noted both the vital role of interruptions and the toll they take. He suggested that "perhaps we can find an ideal middle ground." He then described the work that cognitive psychologist Mary Czerwinski, PhD, did with NASA.

Astronauts monitor the safety of their spacecraft while attending to multimillion-dollar experiments. They need warnings that catch their attention but don't disrupt their focus. Text-filled screens might go unnoticed, but a horn blast could shatter their concentration. So Dr. Czerwinski proposed a visual geometric shape whose sides changed color depending on the type of problem it was signaling. Her solution serves to illustrate Thompson's "middle ground"—and an astronaut's focus zone.

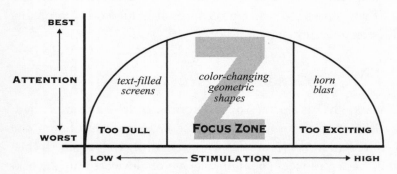

An Astronaut's Focus Zone

Think about the upside-down U curve. A text-filled screen is not activating enough, so the astronaut's response would fall on the understimulated side. A horn blast would trigger too much adrenaline and startle the astronaut into the overstimulated extreme. But the color-changing geometric shape keeps the astronaut in a relaxed-alert state. Astronauts can respond to the warning yet remain in their focus zone.

Personal Control

Here on earth, we usually don't get to choose the shape and color of our interruptions. But we can choose to manage ourselves and our environments, including many aspects of our interruptions. We too can remain in our focus zone.

The keys you learned in Part II will help you deal with interruption. For instance, you can use your assertiveness-skills key to set limits and say no, or your self-talk key to direct yourself back to work. Healthy habits help, too. For instance, by living clutter-free, you create a workspace that makes it easier for you to handle the unexpected.

Your anti-anxiety keys help you to deal with the person who interrupts you the most: *you*. Imagine you're at a meeting and you start to worry about something, which interrupts your concentration. Because you're not paying attention, you won't remember what was said. Later on, you'll worry about what you missed and feel even more anxious and less attentive. By practicing your anti-anxiety skills, you can stop that spiral and restore your attention.

Using your keys gives you a sense of personal control, which you need in order to sustain your focus after you've been hit by stress. Without it, you might handle an interruption while it's happening, but later on you'll pay the price.

In 1971, David Glass, PhD and his colleagues demonstrated how this happens by having college students solve problems in a room with unpredictable, intermittent noise. Students in one group were told they could stop the noise with a signal but were asked not to use it, and they didn't. Another group had no way to stop the noise. During the twenty-four minutes of noise, the two groups performed equally well. It appeared that both groups had adapted to the noise. But then the subjects were taken to another room and asked to proofread under quiet conditions. This time, a significant difference emerged. The subjects who could control the noise in the previous setting now performed much better and showed no tension. The subjects who had no control before now performed poorly and showed a high level of tension. *The critical difference was a sense of personal control.*

Having at least some sense of control matters. If you can control nothing else around you, you can still have self-control. That way, you won't get depleted quickly, like Glass's subjects in the no-choice group. You'll keep enough juice to preserve your focus so you can go on working and still be able to deal with your next interruption.

Plan Your New Beginnings

Another way to exercise personal control is to choose the most strategic time and place to start a project. Research shows that you're more likely to get back into a project if you've already gotten it well under way. In the language of physics, you've gathered momentum. When you need to begin a new project, check your schedule and create a sizeable block of uninterrupted time so that you can get a solid start. It may even be worth an extra trip to the office when no one else is around.

How Do You Recover from Interruption?

According to Thompson, 40 percent of the time, workers wander off in a new direction when the interruption ends. (This helps to account for why it takes twenty-five minutes to get back to your pre-interruption task.) One reason is a lapse of short-term memory: you forget what you're supposed to be doing. Another is motivational: you don't want to remember.

How do you recall what you were working on before you got interrupted? Do you keep your 3-item to-do list directly in your field of vision? Or do you use Post-its with immediate reminders around the edge of your computer screen? Interruptions today are so frequent that organizational experts recommend routinely using some method to keep your current work visible, right in front of you.

Early Adopters

Dr. Czerwinski later worked at Microsoft, where she noticed that many people had attached two or three monitors to their computers. They could place different applications on each screen— for instance, their e-mail program and an open browser off to the side—but keep their main work on its own monitor, right in front of them. These workers reported feeling calmer and believed they were getting more done.

Then Dr. Czerwinski decided to test the effects of more screen space. She asked fifteen volunteers to complete tasks that required concentration on a fifteen-inch monitor and then on a forty-two-inch screen. Productivity increased dramatically. Apparently the tech workers with multiple monitors had instinctively understood the value of having more screen space.

Think about what it's like when you clean out a closet. The more stuff you own, the more open space you need to sort it all out. *The mind needs space to organize and select what's most important* in any visual field—a room, a printed page, or a computer screen. In addition, extra monitor space keeps all your work directly visible, so you can jump right back into it after you've been interrupted.

Tech workers are early adopters—the first to pick up on new gadgets and techniques. I found the idea of using two monitors on a tech worker's blog, years before I'd read about the research on screen space. Then, when I set out to write this book, my husband gave me a nineteen-inch flat screen to use as a second monitor. Now, I'm a big fan. Research is easier, and so is revising, because I can see my source document while I write. I have the same number of interruptions as before, but having all my work in progress just a glance away gives me a sense of control. I can take a call, use my second screen to deal with the interruption, and then sit right down and reenter the action on my main screen—like a movie I just took off pause.

Simplify

At the Emerging Technology Conference in 2004, technology writer Danny O'Brien introduced the term "life hacks" to describe what he called the "tech secrets of overprolific alpha geeks"—the elite of early adopters. He observed, "Geeks have about an eighteen-month lead on trying to find solutions." For example, they were e-mailing and then later dealing with spam about a year and a half before the rest of us. So O'Brien asked top technologists to describe the tips and tricks that they use every day to get things done.

What he found is that productive people often use simple methods. Instead of entering their reminders into complex self-management software programs, they choose a trouble-free text program such as Word or Notepad and type out all the things they have to do and remember.

After the conference, interest in life hacks continued. On his productivity site, 43folders.com, Michael Mann introduced and popularized the "Hipster PDA"—a stack of index cards on which you write all your self-reminders, but which must be small enough to fit into your hip pocket.

It appears that in the future, as technologies grow ever more complex, by necessity, our strategies have to be simple.

TIPS
To Handle Interruption

➤ Use blocks of uninterrupted time to start important projects.

➤ Stay aware of how much of the interruption is work and how much is a break.

➤ Keep a visual reminder of what you are doing directly in front of you so you can return immediately after an interruption.

➤ Use your assertiveness-skills key to limit unhelpful interruptions.

➤ Use your self-talk key to direct yourself to get back to work.

Continuous Partial Attention

In 1998, Linda Stone, a former executive at Apple and Microsoft, coined the term "continuous partial attention." Although most people now use it as a synonym for multitasking, Stone explains that the two concepts are different. In multitasking, you're motivated by a desire to be more productive and efficient. In Stone's continuous partial attention, you're motivated by a desire to be a "live node on the network." You're constantly scanning to make new connections with the best opportunity of the moment.

Stone says that continuous partial attention is neither good nor bad. It just is. It's helpful in some situations, and a hindrance in others. She observed that Bill Gates would have three types of meetings: free-for-all, mixed (sitting at the back indicated paying half-attention), and full (if you're at the table, you focus on what's going on).

Pumping Adrenaline Can Help or Hurt

Most technology conferences today have an Internet Relay Chat (IRC) back channel open as presentations are taking place. Audience members with laptops silently chat about the speaker, spin-off topics, other conference events, or where to meet for dinner. In addition, bloggers blog, often uploading their reviews of the speaker before a talk is finished. This state of continuous partial attention in the audience pumps adrenaline into the moment. With the upside-down U curve in mind, you can see how this could help or hurt. It might boost your energy or make you lose your train of thought, depending on your current adrenaline level and what you need to be in your focus zone.

In my practice, I've seen gifted students who are bored in a traditional classroom, but excel with distance-learning projects in which they watch a video of the speaker and a PowerPoint presentation, chat on a back channel, and build a wiki (Web page that is a collaborative effort by many users). By hopping from one activity to the next, the student stays alert and fully participates in the lesson. Confucius is reputed to have said, "Tell me and I will forget; show me and I may remember; involve me and I will understand."

On the other hand, the college students in my practice who have a fear of missing out (FOMO) don't need any more adrenaline. These hardworking, overextended, sleep-deprived students remain in a state of continuous partial attention because they're afraid to miss an opportunity. It's understandable why they have a feeling that "it could happen at any time." With their always-on communication, they could get a text, instant message, or customized ring on their cell phone any day, anytime, anywhere.

Unfortunately, these hypervigilant students are caught in the same trap as anyone else who lets fear make his decisions for him. They're no longer in charge; their adrenaline is. Eventually, if they don't stop, they will burn out. Continuous partial attention may be continuous, but it is not sustainable.

Unfinished Work Drains You

Interruptions eat up mental energy and stamina. You're doing one thing but still holding a place mark for the thing you didn't finish doing. In addition to Stone's original definition, the term "continuous partial attention" also describes the fragmented, preoccupied state that results from carrying too much unfinished stuff in your head.

This problem is aggravated by the "Zeigarnik effect": people remember uncompleted or interrupted tasks better than completed ones. Bluma Zeigarnik was a Russian psychologist, who noticed that waiters remembered a long, complicated order until they finished serving it.

When you're interrupted or you've got too many irons in the fire, all your "unfinished orders" remain at some level of active mode in your brain. As David Allen, author of *Getting Things Done*, observes, we're conditioning our brains to neither entirely remember things nor entirely forget them either.

Possibly the surest way to recapture a lost sense of personal control is to finish something you've begun. Remember the strategy of adding a super-easy task to your 3-item to-do list? The dopamine boost you get from finishing a task keeps you humming in your focus zone. If you need to free some of your mental energy, find something you can finish right away.

Connected to Life

On July 5, 2006, Thomas Friedman wrote a powerful column for the *New York Times*, "Age of Interruption." In the Peruvian Amazon rain forest with no Internet or cell phone service, Friedman was totally disconnected for four days. He described Gilbert, his guide, who "carried no devices and did not suffer from continuous partial attention." In fact, Friedman reported, "just the opposite." Gilbert heard "every chirp, whistle, howl or crackle in the rain forest" and would immediately identify its source. In Friedman's words:

He . . . never missed a spider's web, or a butterfly, or a toucan, or a column of marching termites. He was disconnected from the Web, but totally in touch with the incredible web of life around him.

Fascination is a powerful antidote for the momentary boredom that the absence of interruption may bring. As Henry Miller once observed, "The moment one gives close attention to anything, even a blade of grass, it becomes a mysterious, awesome, indescribably magnificent world in itself."

Are We Entering the Age of Discernment?

To stay in charge of our interrupt-driven lives, we need effective ways to prioritize. In *First Things First*, Stephen Covey offers one thoughtful solution: categorize all tasks as important, urgent, neither, or both, and make time to act on important tasks, not just urgent ones.

Linda Stone sees a trend toward prioritizing as a natural movement. She believes that the times we're living in are forcing us to ask ourselves, "What do we really need and want to pay attention to?" We're coming to realize that attention is our scarcest and most valuable resource and that what we do with our attention defines us.

Stone says that this puts us on the cusp of an era of "discerning opportunity." Instead of scanning for any opportunity we might miss, we'll filter for opportunities that have the most personal meaning. In this new era, Stone concludes, "engaged attention is to feel alive."

Whether or not this is the future we're all headed for, it's certainly a future to hope for. It would mean that we're living in our focus zone. Relaxed-alert would replace hyperalert, and just-right stimulation would replace the endless quest for more and more stimulation. And unlike continuous partial attention, engaged attention—being in your focus zone—is sustainable over time.

TIPS

To Manage Continuous Partial Attention

➤ Use mindful multitasking to stay in your focus zone.

➤ Act, don't react, when electronic devices summon you.

➤ Stand up to fear of missing out (FOMO).

➤ Don't let unfinished tasks pile up.

➤ Spend time practicing engaged attention.

Use Your Keys to Outsmart Overload

Digital-age data allow you to conduct extensive research; locate people and businesses and contact them instantly; shop in your pajamas; and entertain yourself endlessly with music, photos, videos, games, and interactive media. But the relentless flow of unfiltered information requires you to sift, sort, and select continually, and this makes it a constant challenge to stay in your focus zone. According to an analysis done at the University of California, Berkeley, of the storage and flow of media, the world produced five exabytes of information in 2002. (An exabyte equals 1 billion gigabytes or 1 quintillion bytes.)

If you were startled by the word "exabyte," remember that not so long ago the word "gigabyte" was unfamiliar. And if the amount of new information continues to grow at its rapid current rate—it doubled in the three years between 1999 and 2002—our vocabularies will soon expand as they did from megabyte to gigabyte, onward to terabyte, petabyte, and exabyte.

It's hard to get your head around numbers like these. What point of reference in your everyday life do you have for a number like an exabyte? If just thinking about it starts to jam your circuits, you are experiencing a state of overload that goes by many names. Here are some of them.

Information Anxiety

Richard Saul Wurman coined this phrase. Wurman, an architect and graphic designer, also coined the term "information architecture" to try to bring order to the digital landscape by applying principles of building construction and design.

Information Fatigue Syndrome

Symptoms include forgetfulness, tiredness, irritability, indecisiveness, a shortened attention span, and a lack of concentration. Information fatigue syndrome is the name given to the findings of a report by Reuters titled "Dying for Information." Survey results for 1,300 senior and junior managers indicated that half of these executives frequently or often cannot cope with the volume of information they receive; almost half report that it distracts them from their main responsibilities; and 38 percent waste substantial time because of it. Interviews and focus groups revealed that information overload causes a hyperaroused condition in which executives make "foolish decisions and flawed conclusions."

Analysis Paralysis

What happens when you have too many choices? Your brain freezes, and so you choose none of them. In the Reuters study, 43 percent of the respondents said that their decisions were delayed or adversely affected by analysis paralysis or the existence of too much information. In *Data Smog*, journalist David Shenk describes how the psychological reaction to an onslaught of information and competing expert opinions is simply to avoid coming to a conclusion. In Shenk's words, it "freezes us in our cerebral tracks." Social psychologist Robert Cialdini, PhD, further explains, "You can't choose any one study, any one voice. . . . So what do you do? . . . You don't do anything. You reserve judgment. You wait and see."

Info-Mania

In a recent study conducted in the United Kingdom, eight British workers were given tests of their problem-solving abilities in quiet conditions and in a busy office setting with incoming e-mails and calls. They suffered a sizeable decline in mental sharpness even though it was not their responsibility to answer these messages. Also, as part of the study, 1,000 workers were surveyed. Results showed that 62 percent of adults check work messages after office hours and on weekends, and half reply to an e-mail immediately or within sixty minutes. Another interesting result: while 20 percent said they are happy to interrupt a business or social meeting to respond to a call or e-mail, 89 percent found it rude for colleagues to do so. The term "info-mania" was coined to describe the loss of mental acuity and the addictive tendency that appears to accompany always-on technology.

Attention Deficit Trait

In an article in *Harvard Business Review* (January 1, 2005)— "Overloaded Circuits: Why Smart People Underperform"— Edward Hallowell, MD, identified a "neurological phenomenon" that he called "attention deficit trait." In response to a hyperkinetic environment, when a worker tries to deal with more input than is humanly possible, the brain and body get locked into a reverberating circuit. Hallowell, a psychiatrist, observed that "the brain's frontal lobes lose their sophistication, as if vinegar were added to wine." Symptoms include black-and-white thinking; difficulty staying organized, setting priorities, and managing time; and a constant low level of panic and guilt. In their best-selling book, *Driven to Distraction*, Drs. Hallowell and Ratey called this emerging problem "pseudo attention deficit disorder."

Having read about overstimulation in *Find Your Focus Zone*, you now understand that all these unhealthy, unfocused reactions are signs of being on the overwhelmed side of the upside-down U curve. They signal the kind of cognitive overload that doomed the little donkey in Chapter 3.

These signs can be reframed as cues to take action. To deal with overload, use whatever keys you choose to reduce your stimulation and get back into your zone. Here are some tips to get you started.

TIPS

To Deal with Getting Overwhelmed by Overload
When It's Happening

➤ Four-corner breathing (change-of-state keychain).

➤ An immediate power break (change-of-state keychain).

➤ Set limits and say no (assertiveness-skills key).

➤ Make a plan (anti-anxiety keychain).

➤ Concise, repeated self-direction, "What do I do next?" (self-talk key).

TIPS

To Prevent Getting Overwhelmed by Overload
Before It Happens

➤ Set limits on demands and stimulation (assertiveness-skills key).

➤ Be decisive: aim for good decisions, not perfect ones (sustainability-tools key).

➤ Keep your workspace clear and ready to handle overflow (living clutter-free key).

Mental Filtering Is Necessary

If you're like most people, two main sources of unfiltered information push you out of your focus zone every day at work: e-mail and the Internet. Effective filtering pushes you back in. When you make a strong habit of mental filtering as you go, you harness the unprecedented power that technology provides. You give yourself an edge.

It's smart to use electronic tools—spam filters, pop-up filters, selective RSS feeds, etc.—but even the best software can't do your mental filtering for you. You need an active mental filter to keep you in your zone.

Your self-awareness and stay-on-track keys will help you to exercise your mental filter. Your observer self will keep you honest about the amount of time you're spending online and what you're getting in return. And directive self-talk will keep you on-task, especially when you're tempted by digital diversions.

To mentally filter, start by making a set of rules for what you'll let in and what you'll keep out. Decide specifically what you want and what you don't want to pursue. In the words of an ancient Okinawan proverb, "He who chases around many rabbits ends hungry."

Taming E-Mail

According to the Berkeley study, 31 billion e-mails were sent in 2002, a figure that would double in 2006. A survey by Microsoft revealed that in 2005, the average worker in the United States received fifty-six e-mails per day. At just two minutes per message, that adds up to nearly two hours of time to read and reply. Linda Stone calls e-mail an "attention chipper shredder."

E-mail provides new opportunities to communicate in the workplace—within the office, business-to-business, and business to consumer. And it opens new possibilities for family and friends to communicate across the miles in words and photos. Sitting alone at your keyboard, you feel as if you're sharing your thoughts directly with another person. You can easily forget about the subtle signals you are not sending—the expression on your face, the tone of your voice. Keep in mind that e-mail is a different kind of connection than face-to-face or voice-to-voice contact, and that e-mail is a choice.

One reason for too much e-mail is that it costs nothing—except your attention—to send or receive one. But most e-mail is motivated more by immediacy than cost-effectiveness. Its immediacy is a major reason for you to be self-aware when using it. From time to time check your sent folder for e-mail dated about a month ago. How much of it was more impulsive than worthwhile?

At the end of the day, it's easier to empty your voice mailbox than to get your e-mail to zero. One reason is that e-mail is more permanent. We're generally more careful about what we put in writing to certain people. Another is sheer volume. We get e-mails that were sent to multiple recipients and we are copied on other people's e-mails.

It helps to learn the tips and tricks of your e-mail program and tailor them to meet your own needs. For example, if you frequently use the same sentence or two, save it as a signature so you can insert it with a single click.

It also helps to remember that e-mail is convenient but is not always advantageous. In fact, some companies, such as Nestle Rowntree in Britain, have begun e-mail-free Fridays to see if face-to-face discussions will increase creative problem solving.

Keep your mental filter active when you e-mail. Remember, *what you give your attention to will grow*. Keep your own e-mails clear and concise, and reward your respondents for doing the same.

TIPS
To Tame Your E-mail

➤ Use a reliable spam filter.

➤ Answer noncrisis e-mail at defined times each day.

➤ Be brief.

➤ Stick to core issues.

➤ After you reply, deliberately choose when to send.

➤ Ask yourself "What am I *not* doing now?" (self-awareness key-chain).

Extreme E-mail

In the last several years, wireless handheld devices have been making a cultural impact. On a handheld, you typically receive e-mails as soon as they are sent, so you get more of a stimulant jolt. Heavy users acknowledge that it is often a compulsion, and they experience withdrawal if they stop. It's become a common occurrence at business meetings to see someone's head bowed, glancing downward, in what's known as a "BlackBerry prayer."

When Paul Levy, CEO of a large Boston hospital, revealed in his blog (December 18, 2006) that he was a CrackBerry addict but he'd gone cold turkey that day, he hit a nerve. His blog was picked up by many other blogs, including Tailrank and NetworkWorld. All over the Internet, other CrackBerry addicts admitted ignoring family members, faking excuses with friends, or just being rude so they could read and write e-mails.

Just one week before Levy's posting, the *Wall Street Journal* (December 8, 2006) looked at the same problem from a different angle—through the eyes of children who are frustrated, resentful, and scared because their parents lie, sneak, and ignore them in order to use their BlackBerries. These BlackBerry orphans are jealous of the devices that have taken their parents' attention away from them. One nine-year-old is fearful because his dad types when he drives. "It makes me worried he's going to crash. He only looks up a few times." His dad, a private banker, said it was "a legit concern," but that "some e-mails are important enough to look at en route."

Having read in Chapter 3 how we build up a tolerance for stimulants, you can see how easy it is to get caught in this self-perpetuating cycle. The more dependent you become on your wireless device for day-to-day stimulation, the harder it is for you to be objective about this. It's human nature to justify its importance so as to avoid the discomfort of withdrawal.

If you have a sense that this is happening to you, give some serious consideration to mindful multitasking. Use the keys you've learned, especially your observer self, to begin to break away. Reframe withdrawal as a personal challenge for you to live up to, not avoid. And practice your assertiveness skills and self-talk to set rules for yourself, especially with your family and in your car.

Surfing the Web

New information is posted on the Internet constantly. By the time you've seen all that interests you, more that interests you is already there. Broad bandwidth and HTML e-mail make it easy to get pulled into unintentional, bottomless browsing. A friend sends you a link. That site has several more links of interest. With no waiting time, why not click on those links, and the links they lead to as well?

The Dorito Syndrome

Like Doritos, Internet browsing can be irresistible. You can spend too much time at a task that has no tangible benefit and leaves you with feelings of dissatisfaction and mental bloatedness. That's why early Internet users called browsing a Dorito syndrome. Think of how you feel when you finally get up from your desk if you've lost track of time sightseeing in cyberspace. As with eating empty calories, the minutes are gone; and, instead of feeling satisfied from a nourishing meal, you feel lethargic and sorry you ate the whole bag of chips.

To understand why this happens, recall that when you sat down to browse, you started out hungry, just as you do when you grab a bag of salty chips. You were at the underactivated extreme of the upside-down U curve, and you wanted some stimulation—the latest news or the funniest new video.

Then, as you clicked from link to link, you jumped directly into the other extreme of the inverted U—distracted, indecisive, and overstimulated. In that state it's harder to close your browser window than it is to stop eating chips. At least with chips, you eventually reach the end of the bag.

The pitfall of Internet browsing is that in bouncing from one end of the upside-down U to the other, you skip right past your focus zone. You get up feeling full but not nourished, and even thirstier than before. When you set your mental filter for browsing, make a rule to allow only nutritious information to get in.

TIPS

Sensibly Surfing the Web

➤ Set a time limit.

➤ Keep a clock in view.

➤ Ask yourself "What am I *not* doing now?" (self-awareness key-chain).

Internet Searching

In *The World Is Flat,* Thomas Friedman observed that Google is now processing roughly 1 billion searches a day, up from 150 million just three years ago. Internet searching connects us to a mother lode of useful information, but most web searches yield well over 1 million matches. As Richard Saul Wurman observed, "The opportunity is that there is so much information; the catastrophe is that 99 percent of it isn't meaningful."

Often what starts out as a purposeful Internet search turns into a meandering browse. It's like going to the grocery store for bread and milk, getting attracted to the impulse items at eye level on the end-of-aisle displays, and coming home with the slickest new products—and a bag of Doritos—but no bread and milk. Some early adopters have even written software scripts, such as Webolodean, that pop up every fifteen minutes and prompt you to type in the subject of your search as a forced reminder to stay on task.

It helps to get to know your browser's features. Utilize tabs and keep your bookmarks organized. Rename generic bookmark folders to meet your own individual needs. Instead of folder names such as "Channels" or "News," create specific folders such as "New Car Purchase" or "Lo-Carb Recipes."

It's also useful to learn to search more efficiently. Narrow your searches by entering precision keywords and putting quotation marks around specific phrases. Use commands such as "and," "or," and "not." Read the help centers on search engine sites such as Google for more tips.

To set good rules for mental filtering as you search, start with common sense and then learn from your experience. Here are a few ideas that can help.

Does It Hum or Buzz?

How can you identify high-quality information? One place to start is by screening your sources. Web sites from credentialed individuals, universities, and other noncommercial organizations have less reason to push an opinion that promotes a product or service. But even information from reputable sources can be confusing and often contradictory.

For example, consider the British study on info-mania that I described earlier in this chapter. A number of major news outlets covered the release of the findings. Here's a sampling.

NEWS COVERAGE OF INFO-MANIA STORY			
SOURCE	**HEADLINE**	**LEAD**	**STORY**
London Times	"Why Texting Harms Your IQ"	"The regular use of text messages and e-mails can lower the IQ more than twice as much as smoking marijuana."	"Eighty volunteers took part in clinical trials on IQ deterioration."
CNN.com	"E-mails 'Hurt IQ More Than Pot'"	"Workers distracted by phone calls, e-mails and text messages suffer a greater loss of IQ than a person smoking marijuana."	"80 clinical trials"...

As I read through the reports, I was puzzled. The results added useful information to the field, but the phrasing seemed exaggerated and sensationalistic. The conclusions were worded more recklessly than the way in which a behavioral scientist would speak. Five months later, a blogger provided a more accurate picture of the study.

Apparently, Mark Liberman, PhD, the phonetician at the University of Pennsylvania who runs the Language Log, had the same questions about the study that I had. He wrote a series of posts that came to the attention of the psychologist who had conducted the research, Glenn Wilson, PhD. Wilson explained that his study had two parts: a survey of 1,000 workers and an experiment with eight subjects who tried to solve matrices-type problems with incoming e-mails and calls.

Said Dr. Wilson to Dr. Liberman:

> This, as you say, is a temporary distraction effect—not a permanent loss of IQ. The equivalences with smoking pot and losing sleep were made by others, against my counsel, and 8 subjects somehow became "80 clinical trials."

Hype Buzzes; Facts Hum

In the info-mania story, when I read that the tests used were matrices-type problems, I understood how the hum was turned into a buzz, probably by well-meaning journalists. Matrices-type problems are used in IQ tests. "Temporary Decrease in Problem-Solving Ability" hums. "Loss of IQ Twice That of Smoking Pot" buzzes. The reporters chose the buzz.

Not everything that buzzes is hype, and not everything that hums is fact; but if you hear a buzz while you're looking for an answer, continue to search and listen for a good, steady hum.

It's Eleven-Thirty on Saturday Night

What do you do when it's hum versus hum—when you've found credible data for two sides of an argument? For example, when I was researching jet lag (coming up in Chapter 11), I found a reputable government site that recommended melatonin; but on another site, I found a physician-reviewed article that disagreed. So I hit the medical journals.

I searched for about two hours before I called a halt. A field study showed that melatonin did not help jet lag for 257 Norwegian physicians visiting New York for five days. But a series of studies inside a sleep lab at a medical center showed that it might. I decided to say "conflicting results" and move on.

Whenever I end an Internet search like this, I'm reminded of how Lorne Michaels described the TV show *Saturday Night Live*. In rehearsal, no one ever says, "The show is now as good as it can be; there's nothing more we can do." It's a work in progress until it's time to go on the air live. It's not finished because it's perfect. It's finished because it's Saturday night at eleven-thirty.

The Internet is not going to tell us when it's time to stop a search. We need to stop ourselves. It's up to us to decide when we're finished because it's time for us to "go live" into the real world.

TIPS

For Internet Searching

➤ Name what you're looking for.

➤ Use directive self-talk.

➤ Beware of side trips.

➤ Does it hum or buzz?

➤ Stop yourself. (There's no last page on the Web.)

Defeating Distraction in the 21st Century

The fates lead him who will. He who won't, they drag.
—JOSEPH CAMPBELL, PARAPHRASING THE ROMAN
PHILOSOPHER SENECA

We live in times that challenge our ability to focus. The generations who came before us could not have guessed what it would be like to telecommute to work, conduct e-commerce from a home office, or routinely fly thousands of miles on business trips. Chapter 11 will cover two new high-tech realities of life in the twenty-first century: working from home and working in transit.

Home Office

As technology makes it easier to send data, communicate electronically, and inexpensively share resources, more workers than ever telecommute from home or have started home-based businesses. Nearly 27 million people currently work from home offices, according to research reported by the International Data Corporation.

At home, neighbors can call; kids can need you; the sprinkler system can break; and when you're having a low moment, no one's there to see you turn on Comedy Central and eat ice cream from the carton. You're an island in a sea of distractions.

In a home office, your work setting makes you more prone to

attention swings. It's easy to get bored and understimulated because you are alone without the physical presence of your coworkers. And it's easy to bounce into the overactive side of the inverted U curve with all the intrusions and constantly available diversions—family, friends, pets, chores, and instant entertainment.

If you're considering working at home, first ask yourself these questions:

- ❑ Am I well organized on my own, or do I depend on the organization around me?
- ❑ Is it easier or harder for me to meet deadlines without a buddy or a boss?
- ❑ When I'm alone all day, do I enjoy the solitude or do I feel lonely?
- ❑ Can I say no to distraction during the workday?
- ❑ Can I say no to work when my workday is finished?

If possible, plan a test run before you make a commitment. Talk with others who work from home. Try to find someone who's been satisfied and successful at it and also someone who's decided to return to the office. Which one reminds you more of yourself?

If you are working from home, practice the keys you've learned to stay in your focus zone, especially the 3-item to-do list, power breaks, and mindful multitasking. Adapt these keys for the challenges you face to stay focused in your home office:

- Use the "What am I *not* doing now?" question to stop yourself from getting sidetracked by the comforts and demands of home.
- Make a list of the benefits of working from home. When you get low in motivation and tempted by distraction, read it and reconnect with the reasons you want to work from home.
- Stay clutter-free. File your files and set limits on how many you will stack.

- When you're through for the day, take a cold, hard look at your desk. Leave it in a way that invites you to start working tomorrow morning.
- Use "third space" offices strategically: coffee shops and bookstores if you need more stimulation; the library if you need less.

TIPS

To Set Boundaries between Work and Home

➤ Have a separate, dedicated workspace with a door that closes (not just for tax purposes but for cutting out distraction).

➤ Consider separate e-mail accounts for business and personal use.

➤ Don't answer your home phone when you're "on the clock."

➤ Get up, get dressed, and be at your desk at a set time every morning.

➤ Don't work on your time off, especially on weekends.

Telecommuting

Sheila, an ambitious, hard-driving mother, had a good position in the marketing department of a large company. When another coworker, also a mother, started to telecommute, Sheila thought she should do it, too. Her husband encouraged her, and she submitted a plan to her supervisor that was approved. But almost immediately, it became evident to Sheila that she just couldn't stay focused at home.

When I spoke with Sheila, the reason became apparent. Alone at home all day, Sheila had become preoccupied with the thought that if a promotion became available, she would be overlooked because she was not present. She had been part of her corporate culture long enough to know that her fear was not unfounded.

Sheila was racked with guilt because she felt that, as a mom, she should not give up this opportunity to be at home. Telecommuting was working out fine for her coworker. Why couldn't she do it too?

After a few weeks, Sheila returned to the office. She told me that she realized that she always told her kids to do what's right for them, no matter what someone else was doing. Sheila decided to take her own advice.

Is telecommuting right for you? Weigh all the relevant factors—personal, practical, emotional, and financial. You need a deep, sure level of commitment to your choice so you can resist the distractions that abound at home.

Home-Based Business

Owning your own business provides the freedom to pursue your own goals and make your own decisions. In view of this, it's no surprise that people with ADD qualities (which you'll read about in Chapter 12) are drawn to becoming entrepreneurs. The challenge, of course, is that an attraction to newness—the very trait that can provide an edge—creates problems with maintenance tasks, such as budgets, accounting, inventory, schedules, and allocation of resources.

If you're considering a home-based business, be honest with yourself about your abilities to structure your time, money, goals, plans, and workspace. Are you a visionary who's prone to overlook details? Then use your strengths to troubleshoot the kind of problems that are likely to arise: Join forces with a highly organized partner; hire a virtual assistant; stay accountable to a buddy or spouse. There's no need to deny your vulnerabilities. You're the resourceful type, so it's likely you can tackle your problems, as long as you face them head on.

Shift into your home-based business gradually. Give yourself the chance to practice the tools you need to stay focused. Reach for your stay-on-track keychain:

- Give yourself benchmarks and deadlines.
- Stick to your schedule.
- Keep a clock where you can see it, and use a timer as needed.

Use routines, calendars, planners, and the 3-item to-do list. This also applies if you are home-schooling your child. Structure without pressure is necessary for each of you to stay in your focus zone.

TIPS

For Home Office Workers

➤ Make sure your setup is efficient and ergonomically correct.

➤ Keep calls and e-mails short and on topic.

➤ Post your daily schedule where you can see it.

➤ Review each day's objectives before you begin.

➤ Set the next day's objectives before you leave.

➤ Use your stay-on-track keychain.

Road Warriors

Road warriors of the sky today have to deal with long lines, security hassles, and delays. It's a challenge to stay productive when you're waiting at the gate or cramped in your seat on a plane. The light is dim; air quality is poor; people are talking; babies are crying; and if your plane is late, you're preoccupied with wondering if your connecting flight just took off without you and when you might see your luggage again.

When you're on a business trip, you're functioning at a higher-than-normal level of stress and stimulation. Whether or not you realize it, at a baseline level you're pumping more adrenaline than when you're in your familiar office following your customary routines. Picture the upside-down U curve. At the beginning of your trip, you're on the upper edge of your zone. As your adrenaline burns off, you're at the bottom. Your challenge is to pace yourself and work with the fact that when you're in transit, you constantly have a lowered tolerance for frustration.

Plan Ahead

The best way to stay productive on the road is to plan carefully in advance. In addition to office supplies and items for your personal comfort, ask yourself what you'll need to stay focused in hotels, airports, and planes. Here's a sample checklist:

❑ Earplugs

❑ Earphones (noise-canceling if possible)

❑ A playlist of music to work by

❑ A to-do list especially tailored for being in transit

❑ Treats for breaks and multitasking such as hard candy, chewing gum, and healthy snacks

Educate yourself on the specific hardware and software that suits your needs when you travel. If you're using new equipment or new programs, make time for a dry run before you leave.

"Reduce frustration" is the successful road warrior's credo. Make another checklist of things to do before leaving for the airport. For example:

❑ Download e-mail so you can work off-line.

❑ Fully charge batteries and bring a spare.

❑ Have storage media to back up your work.

❑ Check the TSA Web site for updates on allowable carry-on items.

Keep your checklist with you. That way, when you need some-thing you don't have, you can add it to your list immediately so you'll have it next time.

Create a routine that includes what you pack in your carry-on luggage, what stays with you in your seat, what goes in the overhead bin, and exactly which pouch holds your pens, which one has your glasses, and which one has the boarding pass for your connecting flight. Use the same bag and pack the same things in the same places every time you travel.

When things go wrong, develop self-talk that calms you and keeps you steady:

❑ *Things like this happen on the road.*

❑ *Expect the unexpected; it's part of the adventure.*

❑ *Delays happen to everyone. I'm safe and sound, just late.*

❑ *What positive things can I do with this time?*

Jet Lag

Our bodies have a biological clock that resets our hormones about every twenty-four hours. Jet lag occurs when the body's biological clock does not correspond to local time. It can happen when you travel across several time zones or as a result of shift work.

Symptoms of jet lag include:

- Difficulty concentrating
- Grogginess and loss of mental acuity
- Exhaustion, moodiness, and feelings of disorientation
- Daytime sleepiness and nighttime insomnia
- Anxiety, headaches, and indigestion

Many people use the term loosely to describe feeling tired from traveling, but technically jet lag is a sleep disorder that alters the body's physiology in very specific ways and kicks you out of your focus zone. Unfortunately, the reason you're traveling might require you to be at your sharpest—a world-class competition, a global summit, a military maneuver, a major business deal, or the foreign travel you've saved for all your life.

According to NASA, the more time zones you cross, the longer it takes for you to recover. Exactly how long depends on many factors, including your age, personality, level of physical fitness, amount of preflight sleep debt, and direction of travel. Several studies of flight crews have shown that flying west is easier than flying east.

The evidence for what to do about jet lag is mixed. Most experts agree that it's wise to have some nondrug ways to cope. Sleeping pills are problematic because slowed circulation can contribute to the risk of deep vein thrombosis on long airplane flights, and because even mild hangover effects will add to your grogginess when you wake up. Studies offer conflicting evidence about the effectiveness of melatonin and tryptophan supplements sold in health food stores; both melatonin and tryptophan are produced naturally in the body to regulate sleep-wake cycles. Alcohol worsens jet lag because it disrupts REM (rapid eye movement) or dream sleep, a state that is necessary for sleep to be fully restorative. Caffeine is useful after you land and can drink lots of water, but not in flight when you're prone to dehydration.

Some behavioral approaches are supported by research. They're rather complicated, but if you're very motivated, you might give them a try.

The Argonne anti-jet-lag diet. Developed by the U.S. Department of Energy's Argonne National Laboratory, this diet involves alternating "feast" days of high-protein breakfasts and high-carbohydrate dinners and "fast" days of extremely light eating. A study published in *Military Medicine* showed the diet to be effective with 186 National Guard troops flying across nine time zones.

Light exposure schedules. You can systematically "phase-shift" yourself by increasing your exposure to light and dark, earlier or later each day (depending on the direction you're traveling in). Research at the Rush University Medical Center in Chicago showed that morning intermittent bright light and afternoon melatonin advanced circadian rhythms almost an hour a day. This could be helpful when you're traveling east.

It's possible to borrow the main ideas from these approaches without following them to the letter. For example, if you've just landed in London from New York, bread and potatoes with your dinner might help you later when you're trying to fall asleep. And when your alarm goes off in the morning, you could pull the curtains open right away and drink your tea at a table by the window. If you want to try melatonin when traveling east, the National Institutes of Health suggest one to three milligrams (mg) several hours before bedtime for several nights once you've arrived at your destination.

A practical behavioral drug-free approach is to start to adapt to your new time zone as much as possible a few days before you arrive. Gradually shift the times when you go to bed and wake up. And adjust your exposure to light by using sunglasses and curtains, and by choosing to stay indoors or out.

Several Days *before* You Fly

If you're about to fly . . .	Go to bed and wake up . . .	And choose to . . .
East	Earlier	Seek morning light
		Avoid evening light
West	Later	Avoid morning light
		Seek evening light

If you can afford the time and money, arrive at your destination early enough to adjust, at least one day early, if possible. Elite athletes typically experience less jet lag than most people because of their high level of physical fitness. Nonetheless, they factor jet lag into their schedules because the stakes are so high at world competitions. At the Olympics, serious contenders arrive about a week before their first scheduled event.

TIPS

For Road Warriors of the Sky

➤ Adjust your wristwatch to your new time zone the moment you buckle your seatbelt.

➤ Bring earplugs and an eye mask to help you sleep better.

➤ Drink water; avoid alcohol; use caffeine strategically.

➤ Shift your bedtime and waking time, but do *not* lose sleep.

➤ Give yourself time to recover from travel before important events, and use your self-awareness keychain to prepare for them.

➤ Practice your change-of-state keys to reduce frustration, especially for unforeseen inconveniences.

12

What If You (or Your Children) Have Attention Deficit Disorder?

It is the adaptation to the self that is important,
not the adaptation to the average.

—OTTO RANK

The tools in *Find Your Focus Zone* are for everyone but if you have (or your child has) attention deficit disorder (ADD), you'll benefit from them even more. Learning to use them is a challenge because practice takes patience, which typically isn't your strong suit. But you have other strong suits—you're resourceful and fiercely determined *when you believe in what you're doing.* At this point though, it's understandable that you don't know what to believe about your ADD.

Attention deficit disorder is a relatively new diagnosis steeped in controversy, conflicting data, and a multimillion-dollar support industry. The literal meanings of the words themselves are unhelpful, obnoxious, and untrue: ADD is *not* a "deficit" of attention. People with ADD can concentrate so intensely at times that they are oblivious to the rest of the world. People with ADD have difficulty *regulating* their attention—prioritizing, getting in sync with others, and giving themselves a smooth ride.

Brian, age nine, and his mother arrived at my office for the first time. I noticed the words "attention deficit disorder" in large letters on the cover of the book his mother was reading. I introduced myself to Brian. The first thing he said was, "If you tell me I have that brain disease I'm not talking to you."

The words "attention deficit disorder" seem belittling and offensive to many children and adults. At the same time, if you have this type of brain chemistry, it's useful for you to understand that your brain works differently in some specific ways. When you do, you feel validated. You are free to stop comparing yourself to others unfavorably, and start figuring out how to be your best self. I use the cognitive strategy of reframing ADD—seeing it from helpful yet accurate perspectives—and I encourage adults and children with ADD, and their parents, teachers, and counselors, to do the same. In this chapter you'll learn several specific ways to do this.

What Do You Believe?

If you have ADD, you may be up against the problem that your belief in your ability to strengthen your focus has been shaken to the core. Maybe it's been a rough ride. You've been misunderstood because you don't pay attention the way others do. You pay attention the way you do—you scan and pursue—and this has its upside and its downside.

As you probably well know, when you scan, you don't automatically filter out seemingly irrelevant details. This makes you more likely to spot new ways of seeing things, but also more vulnerable to distraction. And when you pursue, you're prone to get intense, relentless, and extreme. This makes you more likely to persist tenaciously against unfavorable odds, but also more vulnerable to unrealistic ideas.

The downside of ADD causes most adults who have it to continue to carry bad feelings from their childhood days in school. Unfortunately, traditional classrooms are unkind to students who have ADD patterns of focus. Classrooms are set up to reward students who sit still and shut out distractions that come from other kids and from their own imagination and thought processes. And they punish students who do not easily put aside their own pursuits to finish assignments that they regard as too arbitrary and immaterial to their own ideas.

As a child with ADD, did you try to study the way other kids did, but wind up discouraged and frustrated? Were you graded and unfavorably compared with your classmates and siblings? Did you build sturdy walls of self-protection? Did you grow up angry and secretly scared that you were not good enough? Did you create ways to hide your fears from yourself and those around you? *You are not alone, and it was not your fault.*

Frank liked the idea of the 3-item to-do list, but when he tried it, he found he could not choose just three items and let go of the others. All his unfinished work cried out to him as he rushed from one item to another, finishing none. When he forced himself to settle down and be emotionally honest, he realized that his constant sense of urgency was a cover-up for a sinking feeling that he was an imposter.

Frank is highly skilled at computer programming, but deep down, he felt afraid and ashamed that he is a person who promises more than he can deliver. By staying busy with so many projects at once, he diverted his own attention away from his fear and shame. If he slowed down, they surfaced; he felt racked with guilt over past mistakes. As brilliant as he was, he clung to these diversionary tactics, caught in a self-perpetuating cycle. To hide from feeling like someone who doesn't finish what he starts, he stayed busy doing too many things at once; his state of being too busy then caused him to start more things than he finished.

If you, like Frank, start more than you finish, give up your guilt and self-accusations. Instead, understand and appreciate yourself. Consider the many reasons for this pattern in your life:

- People with ADD have an exceptionally powerful orienting response (which you read about in Chapter 3). Your brain is a magnet for novelty; your brain chemistry strongly craves the kind of adrenaline that newness gives you.

- Finishing a project means it's time to get evaluated for it. Most people with ADD grew up with a constant dread of getting assignments returned with lots of red X's for poor grammar, spelling errors, or other details they had overlooked as inconsequential. If you didn't hand in your work, you felt relief because you didn't feel "D-graded." This conditioned you to stop short of completing a job.

- ADD makes you prone to overestimate how much you can do in a given length of time. When you can't keep your promises, you feel guilty, and you hide by jumping into a different activity.

Stay Strength-Centered

After Frank unmasked the constant sense of urgency that both protected and trapped him, he decided to apply an imaginative mental tool that he'd invented for other times when he got too intense and hyperfocused:

I picture what it's like when I drive through the desert in the summer and I see a mirage caused by the heat. The road really does look wavy but I know it's not. Then I remind myself that what I'm doing isn't so urgent after all. It's a mirage caused by how heated up my brain is.

How's that for a handy metaphor to free yourself from the clutches of a fight-or-flight state? This mental tool is exactly right for the job. Using imagery bypasses the need for the brain's CEO to be in charge (which it's not during a fight-or-flight takeover). Imagery doesn't require logic, analysis, or attention to detail. Like Frank, once you recognize buried defenses, you can use your strengths to think up your own imaginative mental tools so you can regain your balance.

New Strategies for Old Problems

No one wants to revisit hurtful memories. Dwelling on pain from the past burns bad feelings more deeply into your brain. But when you trace a defense back to a painful memory and face it, you can free yourself from its grasp and move on.

Learned Helplessness

In the 1970s, psychologists Martin Seligman, PhD and Don Hiroto, PhD conducted a series of studies that showed how early failure causes capable people to quit trying too soon and even lose their ability to learn from feedback. Since then many other researchers have replicated these studies using variations of Seligman and Hiroto's basic model.

In the original learned-helplessness paradigm, subjects had to listen to a loud noise with a button in front of them. For the "escapable noise" group, pushing the button turned off the noise. For the "inescapable noise" group, pushing their own buttons did *not* stop it. They were "yoked" to the escapable-noise group. In other words, for the inescapable-noise subjects the noise stopped when the escapable-noise subjects pushed the buttons. Then each subject was given a new task. To escape the noise this time, all a subject needed to do was move one hand across a "finger shuttle box." The escapable-noise subjects easily stopped the noise this time, as did control subjects who hadn't listened to any noise. But the inescapable-noise subjects did not. Instead, they passively sat and accepted the noise, although the ability to stop it lay at their fingertips. They had learned to be helpless.

In other studies, when three groups of subjects received similar escapable, inescapable, or no-noise conditioning, the inescapable-noise subjects did much worse than the escapable-noise and no-noise subjects on subsequent problems with or without noise. The inescapable-noise subjects did not solve anagrams such as IATOP or find patterns in anagrams when letters were arranged in the same wrong order repeatedly. And they did not benefit from feedback on a card-sorting task to increase the accuracy of predicting their own success or failure.

The responses of the escapable-noise subjects showed that they believed their results depended on their actions. The responses of the inescapable-noise subjects showed that they had difficulty believing their responses could affect success or failure.

When I meet adults who have ADD and they tell me their stories about growing up in school, I am often reminded of the inescapable-noise subjects in the learned-helplessness paradigm. I imagine them sitting in classrooms as children, much as the experimental subjects sat in front of a button that didn't turn off a loud noise. They tried to express their opinions, think for themselves, and pursue questions that mattered to them, but they were misunderstood, reprimanded, and graded poorly.

Now, as adults, they often still feel trapped and unsure that they can succeed. Like the inescapable-noise subjects, they overlook feedback about their new successes and doubt that their responses can affect their own success or failure. Growing up, the only way they could turn off the pain of failure was to stay hidden behind the walls of their defenses. They don't believe that it's different now.

Reframing ADD

ADD is a heterogeneous category that can be viewed from many different perspectives, so why not choose the most helpful one? Get treatment, seek accommodations, and fully utilize resources to help with your ADD, but instead of centering on your weaknesses, *spotlight your strengths.* Reframe ADD for yourself and your child in a way that supports a positive self-image. Some intriguing evidence has been discovered that supports the view that historically, ADD has provided a specific biological advantage.

Hunters in a Farmer's World

In 1993, Thom Hartmann, an expert on ADD, wrote the book *Attention Deficit Disorder: A Different Perception*. He proposed a new view of ADD as a natural adaptive trait: ADD gives you a biological advantage for hunting but a disadvantage for farming. Problems occur when, metaphorically, hunters are forced to farm.

It fits, doesn't it? If you have ADD, you have the same qualities that the best hunters do. You constantly monitor your environment; you can jump into a chase on a moment's notice; and you are capable of sustained drive when you're "hot on the trail." On the other hand, most teachers, librarians, and other people who rule the educational world are more like "farmers." They sustain steady, dependable effort on the tasks of everyday living, and they pace themselves evenly.

In the view of ADD as a disorder, only farmers are normal; hunters are not. In the view of ADD as a biologically adaptive trait, both hunters and farmers are normal. Problems result when hunters clash with the demands of the environment, which, in most situations, currently favors farmers. Here are some more comparisons between the two views.

ADD as a Disorder versus ADD as an Adaptive Trait			
ADD as a Disorder		**ADD as an Adaptive Trait**	
Symptom	Normal	Hunter	Farmer
Inattentive	Attentive	Scanning for game	Focused on chores
Overly intense and urgent	Relaxed	Don't lose that moving target!	Rest at sundown; resume tomorrow
Poor planner	Plans well	What's in front of you right now counts	Anticipate seasons, plant in rows
Impatient	Patient	Cut to the chase; good things move quickly and don't wait for you	Wait for crops to grow; good things take time

In Thom Hartmann's words, "Snap decision making, which we call impulsiveness, is a survival skill if you are a hunter." On the other hand, farming chores have to be done. "If this is a perfect day to plant the crops, you can't suddenly decide to wander off into the woods."

Diversity in Nature Is Good

In January 2002, a group of genetic researchers from the University of California at Irvine reported a remarkable discovery in support of the adaptive trait theory. They were able to trace the first appearance of the gene variation associated with ADD to a point in time 10,000 to 40,000 years ago—and *they demonstrated a positive selection for it* over time. In other words, it had an ongoing advantage to humans.

This gene variation is the 7R allele of the DRD4 gene, which produces receptors for the brain chemical dopamine. (An allele is a genetic unit that allows for variation.) This "novelty-seeking" gene has been linked with ADD and the apparently uneven production of dopamine. The new findings revealed that this variation first appeared during the era when humans were rapidly exploring the earth. On the basis of its significant positive selection, it most likely helped humans thrive and survive. According to Robert Moyzis, PhD, a professor of biological chemistry:

> Our data show that the creation of the 7R allele was an unusual, spontaneous mutation, which became an advantage for humans. Because it was an advantage, the gene became increasingly prevalent. This is very different from other genes that predispose to genetic disorders where the mutations are detrimental.

Does this gene variation continue to be an advantage today? *We are living the answer to that question right now.* Successful hunters are well represented among entrepreneurs, fighter pilots, paramedics, NASCAR drivers, and traders on Wall Street. But less fortunate hunters struggle to succeed in traditional classrooms, office cubicles, and relationships in which they are poorly understood.

Ben was a high school student who had ADD. He got low grades i.. his academic subjects at school. Although his teachers liked him, they regarded him as a poor learner.

One summer, Ben went to China on a study-abroad program. While there, he put his heart and soul into experiencing China as if he were Chinese. He worked in fields and factories, made friends, tried to speak Chinese, and used chopsticks; and when families offered him dishes made with turtles, frogs, or fish heads, he tasted whatever they served him. The other students in the program ate out at McDonald's instead.

Outside the classroom, Ben is actually a much better learner than most people. He didn't memorize facts about China from books. He was a true student of China, breathing it in and making it part of him.

Living with the 7R variation of the dopamine gene *will become what we make it*. It's up to us to understand and appreciate its worth. Biological diversity is one of Mother Nature's greatest gifts to us. Hunters and farmers alike can benefit by remembering that *any strength carried to excess is a weakness*.

At the invitation of a friend, I once attended a meeting of an investment club that had been inspired by the famous "Beardstown ladies." This particular group of women happened to be thorough, meticulous, and methodical. They intelligently researched and discussed analysts' ratings, expense ratios, earnings per share, growth rate measures, net asset values, alpha, beta, volume, and volatility of various stocks. But several hours later when the meeting adjourned, they still hadn't made a single purchase. The phrase that kept going through my mind was "farmers in a hunter's world."

Susceptibility Genes

It also helps to understand another important aspect about the genes that are linked to ADD. Genes that influence attention are *not* the same as genes that determine the color of your eyes. Geneticists call dopamine receptor genes such as DRD4 "susceptibility" genes. In other words, they interact with other genes and the environment to create a "potential" for ADD. Biology is *not* destiny when it comes to traits such as human attention.

According to geneticists, hundreds of genes influence our individual personalities, and evidence points to a continuum of traits. In other words, attention disorders are the extreme of a normal range of aptitudes and qualities. Your other genes, the skills you've learned, and your current work setting all contribute to whether or not you have ADD and how severe it is if you do.

Let's say you do have the 7R allele of the DRD4 gene and you produce dopamine unevenly. You might also have other genes that mitigate its effects, such as those that influence serotonin production. Or your dad may have had the same gene and taught you at a young age how to deal with it, perhaps by his good example. Maybe you work in a setting that doesn't require a lot of "farming" chores. *You could have the traits that come with the gene but not the severity of problems that make it a "disorder."*

The Edison Trait

In my first book, I described the personality profile of bright, imaginative people who are "divergent thinkers." In other words, their minds spark with many ideas at once in a nonlinear popcorn-popping way. Unlike "convergent thinkers," whose minds are sequential and orderly, Edison-trait adults and children often collide with the outside world.

> Sophie, now a college sophomore, came to my office laughing one day. When I asked her why, she said that she had just passed by her junior high school at dismissal time and many of the kids had rolling backpacks. She explained that when she was in the seventh grade, she had gotten one to take to school. As in many schools today, students couldn't have lockers (so they can't hide contraband). As a result they have to carry all their heavy textbooks with them to and from school. When Sophie brought her

rolling backpack to school, she was ostracized for being "odd." Now, it turns out that she was simply ahead of her time.

Sophie had seen an original, resourceful solution that no one else saw; this is a definitive characteristic of the Edison trait. This penchant for divergent thinking was named for Thomas Edison, who was so nonconforming that he got kicked out of school twice. When Edison was taught in a way that emphasized his strengths—encouraged to build his own science lab so his inquisitive mind could flourish—he became the most prolific inventor in the history of the United States.

If you have Edison-trait characteristics, you're more likely to have ADD. This makes it all the more important for you to practice skills and strategies to stay in your focus zone. As you may recall from Chapter 4, your habits over time strengthen or weaken specific pathways in your brain.

Be like Thomas Edison and use your strengths to face your challenges. The habits you practice make the difference in your success. *Genes don't determine human behavior; the choices you make do.*

Your Focus Zone Is Surrounded by Cliffs

People who've developed good strategies to cope with the challenges of ADD often hold onto them with all their might.

- *"You don't understand. I have to clean up my desk before I go to bed. I'm not like everyone else. If I leave it messy, I won't be able to sit at it for days."*
- *"For some people, exercise is exercise. If they miss it, they make it up. For me, exercise is everything. If I miss it, my day is shot."*
- *"When I work, I put my cell phone in another room. Turning it off just isn't enough. I'm like a chocoholic who's got to keep anything chocolate out of reach and out of sight."*

If you have ADD, when you get distracted, you have to fight your way back to getting focused again. So once you find a routine that works, you are wise to stay with it even if others wonder why you're being so particular.

Think of the upside-down U curve. Picture the arc that goes up from bored to focused and down from focused to hyper. For most people this gradient is a gentle, gradual slope. For you, it's a high cliff. If you fall off, you've got a steep hike to get back into your zone.

Recognize and Strategize

If you have ADD, you can help yourself by engaging in healthy habits: regular sleep, balanced nutrition, physical exercise, savvy use of stimulants—all the behavior skills you learned in Chapter 8. These routines will help you to stay off the edge of the cliff.

In addition, helpful self-talk lets you work *with* your ADD, not against it.

Recognize: "I cut things close."
Strategize: "I'll leave extra time."

Recognize: "I need the stim."
Strategize: "I'll study at the bookstore."

Recognize: "I need the quiet."
Strategize: "I'll study at the library."

When you reframe your ADD in positive terms, you'll have less of a need to protect yourself. You're freer to recognize the problems for which you need strategies. You can acknowledge your difficulty judging time, for instance, and get better at building in a buffer of time when you've got a due date or an appointment.

Recognize that you have a relationship with stimulation that's different from most people's. Some days you *must* go to the coffee shop to study; you need new sights and sounds, and the infusion of energy that you get from other people's presence. Some days you *must* go to the library. The sound of your own breathing distracts you.

Learn as much as you can about *your* ADD. Recognize that ADD has as many different presentations as there are people who have it. As Carl Jung once said, "All the corpses in the world are chemically identical, but living individuals are not." What matters is what *you* need to do to stay in your focus zone.

Medication: A Personal Decision

All medications to treat ADD help to regulate adrenaline in some way. The most widely used drugs—Ritalin, Adderall, and Concerta—are stimulants that are believed to act on dopamine receptors.

The decision to use medication to treat your ADD, or to treat your child's ADD, is highly individual. Educate yourself and weigh out your concerns. What are the risks? What are the benefits? Talk with your doctor. Explore *all* your choices, drug and nondrug.

Be open to different possibilities. Sometimes two people can have very similar symptoms, but medication is right for one person and not the other. A medication may work well during one phase of your life, but less so just a year or two later. Medication for ADD is a choice you make over and over again as your life changes.

Stimulants are effective within about an hour of taking them, and their effect can last from several hours to all day if you take a sustained-release form. Because of this you can choose how you want to use them as a tool. Many people take medication in some situations but not others. For years I've counseled a writer with ADD who uses medication judiciously. When he has to pay attention to details such as research notes and business accounting, he takes it. When he wants to think freely, make new connections, and write creatively, he does not.

A Tool, Not a Crutch

If you do choose to use medication, the way you think about it matters. Taking medication doesn't mean that you no longer need to practice skills and strategies. It means that you now have a powerful tool to get even better results when you practice them.

If you decide to give medication to your child, how you present it can be crucial. Some parents discover this on the first day they forget to give their child his pill. The child fails a test that he didn't even try to pass, because he remembered that he missed his meds. Or the parents are summoned to school because their child slugged a classmate, explaining that it was "because I didn't have my medicine today."

Let your child know that medication does not replace self-control. Its purpose is to support his efforts, not be a substitute for them. Explain that medication doesn't take the place of building skills and applying strategies. It's a means to help strengthen his ability to build them.

Research shows that 30 percent of the children who take medication for ADD stop taking it within two years, and 60 percent stop taking it within three years. According to the *Educators Manual* of Children and Adults with Attention Deficit Disorder (CHADD), "The implications for over-reliance are clear. Perhaps the use of medication is best viewed as a window of opportunity wherein educators focus on teaching organizational and learning strategies."

Adults as well as children can use the experience of being on medication as a window of opportunity to learn. When you experience what it's like to feel more organized, you have more cues so you can try to feel that way again.

If you have high blood pressure, taking beta-blockers doesn't mean you can eat salty foods or become a couch potato. If you have high cholesterol, taking statins doesn't make fatty foods, creamy sauces, and rich desserts OK. Taking a stimulant for improved attention is no different. For best results, you need to use it in combination with the right program of mental diet and exercise. Continue to practice the skills, strategies, and healthy habits that keep you in your focus zone.

The Bannister Effect

How much of any human limitation is mental, and how much of it is physical? Except for obvious extremes—flying off the top of a tall building—the most correct answer is, "We don't know." And because we are all in a continual state of change, the most empowering answer is, "Give it your best shot and see."

Before 1954, no one had run the mile in less than four minutes. People thought it was medically impossible and that a person's heart would burst from the pressure. Then, Roger Bannister became the first runner to do it. Within a year, many others also broke the four-minute mile. Seeing that it could be done, these runners changed their self-limiting beliefs.

Today, many people with ADD have learned to focus and succeed, some with spectacular results. David Neeleman, founder and CEO of JetBlue and inventor of the electronic ticket, has capitalized on his ADD strengths, which he says far outweigh the problems that ADD has caused for him. Paul Orfalea, founder of Kinko's, used it to his advantage, too. He insightfully objects to the word "deficit" because he doesn't think it is true. A close friend of his calls it "AAD" for "accelerated attention disorder."

If you've come to believe that it's physically impossible for you to break through your barriers—if you have a sense of learned helplessness about them—maybe it's time to question your limits. Like Roger Bannister and all the runners who dissolved the barrier of the four-minute mile, be open to a new belief. In my practice, I've worked with people who've had their own private "Bannister breakthroughs"—sitting in a classroom deciding to give their all to get a higher grade, taking on new responsibilities at work, or recommitting to a relationship with a new willingness to be fully present in it.

Is it time to give yourself a fresh start? As Norman Cousins once observed, "Progress begins with the belief that what is necessary is possible."

Part IV

Your Focus Zone
as a Way of Life

The more you use your new keys, the easier it will be for you to stay in your focus zone and teach your children to stay focused, too. The concluding chapters in Part IV will help you to guide your children, and encourage you to appreciate the power of your attention every day.

13

Teaching Kids to Pay Attention

If the challenge of parenthood can be reduced to one basic task, it is helping children develop their own talents, skills, and resources for coping with life without their parents.

—LEE SALK, PhD

I was giving a talk to parents in which I explain how to help kids make good choices about TV and video games. One mother in the audience spoke up: "I don't understand the big deal about what *the child* decides to do. I decide when the TV goes on and when it goes off and that's that. Don't other parents even have that much control?" I asked her how old her children were. She said they were nine and eleven years old. I realized she had no idea what kind of storm was about to hit her house in the next year or two.

I have counseled hundreds of children, teenagers, and young adults. Their resourcefulness knows no bounds. If they want to see an R-rated DVD, they will; they have friends who watch television unsupervised. If they want to play M-rated video games, they do; they know which arcades look the other way. They may have difficulty researching a history paper, but they can easily find Web sites on how to bypass parental Internet controls and delete the trail of Web sites they've visited. And when they leave for college, those who have lived under the strictest rules at home get drunk with freedom—and lots of beer—every chance they get.

Teenagers and young adults need to test limits. It's in their job description—the developmental task of their age. Think back to your teens and twenties. Did you experiment with choices you wouldn't have made if your parents had been present?

We cannot control our children. They began exercising their free will in their high chairs when they refused to eat the strained vegetables we tried to feed them. *We can teach them self-control.* And then they can make good choices whether we're around or not.

Teaching Seslf-Control

Don't let yourself get caught in control battles, and don't let your child push your buttons. You're the adult. Refuse to be on opposite sides.

This doesn't mean that you "give in." It means reframing your parent-child relationship so that what's most important—even when you disagree—is that you're both on the same side. You can hold the line, be assertive, set limits, enforce rules, and hold your child accountable, all without drama, yelling, or commotion.

Think of the way a police officer pulls you over if you're speeding. The officer doesn't scream at you or ask you how you could do this to her again. In a respectful, matter-of-fact way, she writes a ticket and holds you responsible for your actions.

A parent is a child's first teacher. You are in an excellent position to guide your children to build attention skills, but only if they trust you and feel your support as they stumble through the inevitable mistakes they need to make to learn and grow.

Maturity Matters

The way you teach self-control depends on a child's age. Small children need simple, straightforward rules to follow. Until your child is about age seven, act more; explain less. An easy weekly star chart can be helpful. List your child's three or four most important daily routines, preferably in pictures, with a box for a star or sticker for each day of the week. Remember to include quiet time.

At around age seven, begin an educational approach to teaching self-discipline. Ask yourself what your child is learning from the way you set limits and follow through. Is your child learning to hide the truth from you, to avoid getting punished? Or is your child learning to correct her mistakes so she can improve?

Protect children with rules until they're mature enough to handle matters on their own. As they get older, gradually let them have more say in making the rules they will live by.

Five Steps to Teach Kids to Pay Attention

This chapter describes five steps for teaching children how to stay in their focus zone:

STEPS TO TEACH KIDS ATTENTION

Step 1: Be a good role model.

Step 2: Reward attention, *not* interruption.

Step 3: Give your child tools.

Step 4: Set limits.

Step 5: Believe in your child.

Reframing can help you keep a healthy perspective. If you get infuriated or discouraged, use your feelings as a cue to remind yourself that your son's or daughter's childhood will go by quickly. Look beyond your frustrations and remember to enjoy this precious time. Appreciate yourself, all you do, and the unprecedented challenges you face today as a parent. The demands are great, but the rewards are even greater.

Step 1: Be a Good Role Model

Sarah was an imaginative, daydreaming child, who had problems staying focused on her homework. Psychological and educational testing showed that she was bright but immature and borderline

ADD. Jackie, Sarah's mother, had read my book *Dreamers, Discoverers, and Dynamos*. She came to see me to learn what she could do at home to help her daughter.

I asked Jackie to describe what the house was like while Sarah did her homework. She said that she was in the kitchen cooking, and Sarah was nearby at the kitchen table so she could ask for help. Her younger son, Sam, played in the family room where Jackie could keep an eye on him from the kitchen. Her husband didn't get home from work until seven o'clock in the evening.

When I met with Sarah we talked and drew pictures together. When she got engrossed in her drawing, Sarah reassured me, "It's OK. I'm still listening," although she was not. After the session, when her mother and brother returned, Sarah's behavior regressed as she competed with Sam for her mother's attention.

At my next meeting with Jackie, I had a better understanding of homework time through Sarah's eyes. It started with her role model: her hardworking, well-intentioned, multitasking mother. Sarah didn't see a woman who was concentrating on what she was doing. She saw her frenzied mom, who was jumping from a recipe book to a crying son to a daughter's questions about homework. If Jackie was adding spices, timing a sauce, or watching a boiling pot, and Sarah tried to get her mother's complete attention, Jackie half-listened but reassured her daughter, "It's OK. I'm still listening." And if Sarah asked her a question while Sam was pitching a fit, Sarah learned that the least mature action won Jackie's attention first. Then she whined and cried to get her mother's attention too.

Solving the Problem

Jackie made a new plan for homework time. She changed to dinner menus that required very little immediate attention, and she stopped Sam from constantly interrupting. Sam liked Legos, so Jackie established a routine in which she sat down with him and gave him ten minutes of undivided attention until he got involved in whatever he was building. Then about every ten minutes that

Sam played quietly by himself, she wordlessly dropped a Lego into a clear jar on the counter. When the jar was full, Sam would get the new Lego set he wanted. If Sam interrupted to ask if it was time to put a Lego in the jar, it would take another ten minutes for him to get one. If Sam didn't interrupt for at least half an hour, he could choose a DVD to watch when he was done.

A Focused Role Model

At last, Jackie was free to sit down with Sarah while she did her homework. I had encouraged Jackie to learn more about mirror neurons, which she did by reading *Social Intelligence* by Daniel Goleman. With her new appreciation for the power of modeling, when Jackie sat down with her daughter, she chose work that required concentration—paying bills, balancing the checkbook, catching up with correspondence. Silently, they sat together at the table and focused—Jackie on her work, and Sarah on hers.

Jackie forced herself not to jump up when the phone rang or when she remembered a chore that needed to be done. Her goal was to remain in her own focus zone. *With mirror neurons at work, Sarah would be drawn into her focus zone too.*

When Sarah asked a question, Jackie gave her undivided attention, but she didn't do Sarah's work for her. Instead she returned to her own work, with the unspoken expectation that Sarah would do the same. The feeling in the room was completely different from before. Instead of a noisy state of perpetual motion with no results, the tone was calm and quiet and a feeling of work getting accomplished was in the air.

Soon Sarah began to complete her homework every night and to feel proud of her success. She still daydreamed her way through life—that was her personality. But now when Sarah sat down to do homework, she stayed with it until she finished. Gradually Jackie left Sarah by herself at the kitchen table for longer and longer periods of time. She continued to keep a distraction-free setting and a work-time feeling in the air. And she continued to stay aware of the effect on Sarah—for better or worse—of her own behavior.

Staying Aware

Intellectually, Jackie had known that her own divided attention at dinnertime had been disruptive for Sarah, but she first had to develop enough self-awareness while she was doing it, so that she could change. I've seen families in counseling where everyone interrupts everyone else and everyone knows it, but no one is aware of interrupting at the moment it's happening. How aware are you of what your actions teach your child?

One especially important time to set an example of how to stay focused under pressure is if you have a fender-bender with your children in the car. Your adrenaline is pumping hard and fast and it's a real challenge to keep a clear head. It's also a rare opportunity for them to see what you do when you have a brush with danger. Mentally rehearse how you want to react. See yourself staying calm and in your focus zone. Remind yourself that you're planting the seeds for how they'll react years from now when they're driving and they have a minor accident or they suddenly face danger.

Your observer self will tell you how your growing child sees you. Or your growing child might tell you this. Another parent at a workshop told me his son said, "Daddy, your BlackBerry is like my Game Boy. When is it time for you to put it away?"

It's OK to make mistakes. No one is a perfect parent. In fact, a mistake is a chance to set a good example for what to do when you make a mistake. *A good role model is aware, not perfect.*

Step 2: Reward Attention, *Not* Interruption

When Sarah had a long or difficult assignment, Jackie stayed close by. She wanted to reward Sarah immediately for independent work. She did not want go back to rewarding Sarah only when she got stuck, quit working, and jumped up to get help.

As Jackie washed the fruit or emptied the dishwasher, she quietly kept an eye on her daughter. When she saw that Sarah had just finished a page of problems, or was changing books for her next assignment, Jackie called to her, "Good job, Sarah.

You're really staying with it." Without causing a distraction, she complimented Sarah periodically while Sarah stayed focused on her work.

When Sarah entered the fifth grade, she began to do her homework in her own room. Jackie was worried because now she couldn't see those opportune moments to reward Sarah's perseverance. So she invented ways to look in quietly on her daughter and reward her for staying on-task without also causing a distraction.

Most afternoons, when Sarah had been working for about half an hour, Jackie brought her a simple treat—lemonade or a healthy snack—with a short note: "So proud of you," "You can do it," "Way to go!" or just a flower or a smiley face. Sarah looked forward to her mother's stopping by and didn't let it interrupt her work. It made her try even harder to keep working. She knew this would please her mom, and she could see how hard her mom was trying to please her.

Sarah learned to complete her homework alone in her room. When she needed a break, she took one, so she could stay in her focus zone. But she no longer sought her mother's attention every time she began to lose her own. She learned to keep working and save her questions for later. It was particularly satisfying for Sarah when she did this and then discovered the answer all by herself because she had kept working.

Asking for Trouble

At first it seems counterintuitive to reward a child for paying attention while she's paying attention. You don't want to risk distracting her. You know how hard it was to get her to settle down in the first place. It feels a little like waking a sleeping baby. You're just asking for trouble.

The fact is, you're asking for trouble if you reward a child for *not* paying attention. "The squeaky wheel gets the grease" is true for wooden carts; but when it comes to kids, you'll get louder and more frequent squeaks. If you pay attention to your child only when she gets stuck, she'll get stuck more of the time so she can get your attention. If you stop what you're doing and walk over to her only when she's distracted, you're inadvertently training her to become distracted again.

Effective teachers use the "catch 'em being good" method. When it's time for the class to quiet down and pay attention, they say, "I see Johnny ready to listen," "Mary's ready now, too," "And now Paul, and Linda . . ." These teachers know that the behavior they reward with their attention will occur more often in the future.

Mommy Likes Me Best

Did you ever notice how a young child can be focused on what she's doing; but the moment you answer the phone, she's at your side, focused on you? A parent's attention is an attractive prize, and it's even more attractive when someone else wants it too.

You can help young children by practicing real-life situations with them ahead of time. Ask your child to tell you "a good choice" for her to make when you're on the phone or talking face-to-face with another adult. She might say, "Stay quiet," "Find something to do," or "Stand on one foot so you know I'm waiting for you." Then ask her to show you what it looks like when she makes that good choice, so she actually rehearses doing it. Pretend the phone is ringing, you pick it up, and she makes a good choice. Practice as many times as it takes, and be sure to smile, hug her, and say, "Good job!" This gives you many chances to reward her attention, not her interruption.

Next time the phone actually rings, help her be successful by not making her wait too long. Then shower her good choice with your undivided attention.

Step 3: Give Your Child Tools

Build Your Child's Vocabulary for Attention

Talk with your child about attention. Help her name her moods, mental states, and behaviors. A descriptive label can serve as a useful handle to help her grasp what she needs to do. Use words such as these:

"on-task" or "off-task"

"focused" or "distracted"

"in your zone" or "spaced out" or "hyper"

"your focus zone"

"change of state"

"facing it" or "avoiding"

In my practice, I've worked with many parents who realize that nagging children to keep doing their homework is not effective. In fact, it usually triggers the opposite response. But not doing anything about it isn't effective either.

When parents use this problem as a learning opportunity, they soon see better results. It's a challenge to be nonjudgmental and use an educational approach. In step 3 you'll learn many methods to do this. A good place to start is by teaching your child to develop an observer self and become more aware of what she's doing:

- I see you're *on-task*. Good for you!
- Are you *on-task* or *off-task* right now?
- What can you do to get back *on-task*?

Most kids say "I'm bored" pretty easily. They assume that all they can do is react to what's exciting or dull outside them. Don't be tempted to take responsibility for their boredom. It reinforces the message that there's nothing *they* can do about it.

Do take responsibility for being part of a culture that supports their false assumption by giving them a world of instant entertainment. As adults, it's up to us to teach our children that the center of power lies inside them, not in their remote control.

Let your kids know that they *can* turn things around themselves when they're bored. Remind them of times when they became more involved, engaged, or fascinated and had fun. Ask them, "What can *you* do to make it more interesting for yourself?" or "What's your imagination got to say about that?" When they answer, "I don't know," turn it into a playful game. Once their minds get heated, they will do the rest.

Avoidance versus Taking a Break

Greg and his parents had an ongoing battle about his homework. Almost every night Greg would balk at some part of his assignment, causing a long-drawn-out discussion or a tense, angry fight. Either way, without anyone's realizing it, Greg successfully baited his parents to help him avoid his work.

In counseling, when I brought up the subject of Greg's low grades, he said, "I don't want to talk about that." I validated his feelings of embarrassment and guilt, and told him we could take a break any time he felt overwhelmed. We'd go for a ten-minute walk, and then discuss schoolwork when we got back and he had a better attitude. "We need to face problems, not avoid them," was my persistent positive message—a message that Greg eventually came to trust.

When Greg was willing to stay on-topic for even a few minutes, I let him know he was gutsy for talking about his problems. At home, Greg's parents learned to defuse arguments over homework and recognize how his fights served as avoidance. They could see how adding guilt just made Greg avoid facing it even more. Soon Greg was recognizing his own avoidance.

Kids can't bear the pain of disappointing their parents or feeling like a loser in front of their peers, so they create all sorts of diversionary tactics to avoid the risk of not making the grade. Their avoidance gives them the relief they need, but digs them into a hole. Taking a break also gives them this relief, but gets them back to facing what they're running away from, when they feel a little better. Once Greg, like many other kids, grasped this difference, he began to make steady progress.

As you may recall from reading about power breaks in Chapter 5, the difference between avoidance and taking a break is that *when you take a break, you return to work*. It helps to frame this in terms kids can understand and respect. You don't flake out on yourself, like leaving someone stranded at a mall. You come back to face your problems, because your life matters and you are worth it.

Your Child's Focus Zone

Kids are prone to attention swings, so they usually relate to the concept of the upside-down U curve. Draw them a picture of it. Ask them to point to the place on the curve where they are right now. Draw a Z on the curve, so they can see their focus zone. Help them understand that they can add stimulation when they feel bored, and reduce stimulation when they're in overdrive. Ask them to tell you their ideas and plans for how to do it.

Have your child write down three things he can do to settle down and focus. Do this when he is in his zone, so he'll have the list on hand when he's not. Photocopy it, so it can be handy at home-work time. When something works well, let your child know he came up with a useful idea. When something stops working, reassure him that this is to be expected, and it just means it's time for some fresh ideas.

Practice the change-of-state key with your child. Make it a game. Learning to pay attention doesn't have to be painful. It can be playful and rewarding.

Bad Choice / Good Choice

If your child is inattentive or impulsive, teach him self-control by having him rescript his mistakes. This gives him a chance to learn and feel motivated to do better next time. Let's say he spaced out at school today and forgot to hand in an assignment.

If all you do is reprimand and ground him, what has he learned? Probably to try harder next time to make sure you don't find out.

If you ask him to tell you what he could have done differently, he's likely to start out by saying, "I don't know." But with some coaching, you can help him make a plan so that he'd finish the assignment if he were in the same spot again. Some kids need more help than others; but be careful—it needs to be his plan, not yours. An older child might be ready to start using some self-talk: *"I've done hard things before. I can do this too."* A younger child might need to know he can ask the teacher for help.

In addition to coming up with a plan for next time, have your child finish the assignment and hand it in, even though it's late. Now you can say, "Well done," and reward his efforts to make a better choice and succeed.

The beauty of the bad choice / good choice method is that you give your attention to the things he's doing right, not the thing he did wrong. To use this method:

1. *Identify the bad choice.*
2. *Ask him what a good choice would have been.*
3. *Practice and reward the good choice.*

Children's Self-Talk

When you teach children to use positive self-talk, you give them a gift that lasts a lifetime. A child's brain absorbs language like a sponge.

When a child is not paying attention and then puts himself down, he's forming a habit that limits his success. The earlier you can get him to break this habit, the better. Ask him which he thinks is more helpful for him to say: "I'm stupid," or *"I learn from my mistakes."*

Keep in mind that the things you say to your child become the things he says to himself. Which do you want him to hear in his own head: "You're so forgetful," or *"You can remember. Just calm down and it will come to you"*?

With self-talk, kids of all ages can coach themselves to success. Here is the self-talk of an eight-year-old boy who has made enormous progress staying in his zone both in school and in sports. He came up with this on his own, based on his understanding of his own focus zone. (He likes to call himself by name when he uses self-talk):

"Nick, your adrenaline is up. You're more mature than this and you can do better."

Step 4: Set Limits

Sleep

As early as 1925, research linked sleep and the development of intelligence in children. Lewis Terman, PhD, who originated the Stanford-Binet Intelligence Test, found that in every age group he studied, the longer children slept, the better they performed at school.

Although each child's need for sleep is different, the National Sleep Foundation recommends these guidelines:

- Preschoolers (3 to 5 yrs)—11 to 13 hrs, including naps
- School-age (5 to 12 yrs)—9 to 11 hrs
- Adolescents—8 to 10 hrs

A study at Brown Medical School of six- to twelve-year-olds showed that those students with eight hours or less sleep per night had the most problems paying attention in school. A study at the University of Michigan linked poor sleep with symptoms of attention deficit disorder, especially in boys age eight and under, prompting psychologist Gahan Fallone, PhD, to comment, "Getting them to sleep on time is as important as getting them to school on time."

Kids can get strong-willed at bedtime—the exact time when parents are the most exhausted. But bedtime doesn't have to be battle time. Deal with this issue earlier in the day when you and your child are less tired and more rational.

Decide how much sleep is right for your child. Pick a good time during the day and secure your child's commitment. This may take some ingenuity. Depending on your child's age, appeal to his sense of reason. Think of an incentive to kick-start his new habit. If your child is in bed on time five nights in a row, for instance, he gets to invite a friend for pizza and a movie. After about three weeks, you can fade out the incentives. The new habit will have begun to set in.

Work together to create a bedtime routine that supports your child's success. Start early enough to turn off electronics and tone down the running and jumping around the house. Have a bedtime ritual—soothing music, dim lights, relaxing reading, and saying good night. If your ritual works, stay with it. If not, work together with your child *during the day* to make a new plan.

Tips for helping kids get the sleep they need:

- Establish a regular bedtime for school nights and another for weekends.
- Have a specific time to get ready and another for lights out.
- Limit your child's sugar and caffeine, especially after 2 PM.
- Keep TVs and video games out of the bedroom.
- Make getting enough sleep a family priority, not a control issue.
- Keep bedtime rituals pleasant, peaceful, and loving.

Television and Video Games

In Chapter 9 you read about flicker and the American Academy of Pediatrics' recommendation that children up to two years of age watch no television at all. For older children the academy recommends no more than one to two hours per day of educational, nonviolent programs. It also recommends that TV sets be removed from children's bedrooms.

Children in the United States today watch an average of three to four hours of television per day, not counting movies on DVDs or video games. One study found that children spend an average of six hours thirty-two minutes per day with various media combined. Another found that 32 percent of two- to seven-year-olds and 65 percent of eight- to eighteen-year-olds have TV sets in their bedrooms.

With this kind of gap between the recommendations of experts and the reality of the world today, what happens when you set a limit for your children? They tell you Johnny can watch, Mary's allowed, and Tim has a TV in his room. They enjoy watching and want to fit in. The American Academy of Pediatrics—highly credible, scientifically based, and dedicated to the health and growth of children's brains—just doesn't make the list of what matters most to them. So what can you do?

For preschoolers and children in the primary grades, you decide when the TV is on or off. Say simply, "Because it's quiet time now," "Because it's time for our brains to think," or "Let's go outside and play."

For older children, teach them self-control:

- Watch a commercial with your child and deconstruct it together. Ask him to tell you how the advertiser is trying to make him feel as if he cannot live without the latest electronic toy.
- Be a good role model, and share your thinking without lecturing. When you turn off the TV, let your child know that just like him, you still felt like watching more.
- Tell your child you're proud of his choice when he clicks the TV off by himself.
- Ask your child how much TV he thinks is good for him. Talk in terms of specific hours and minutes, so he learns to keep track of his time.
- Listen to your child's opinions and ask "Socratic questions" tailored to his specific interests: "I wonder how much TV an astronaut has time to watch. What do you think?"
- Have other, nonelectronic forms of entertainment readily available—a musical instrument, cool games and puzzles, books of jokes and comics.
- Bring in experts your child cares about—discuss the issue together with his own pediatrician at his next checkup.

Continue to have rules, such as no TV until homework is done. But let children have input on leisure-time rules to the extent that they can handle it responsibly.

When it comes to teenagers and video games, stay involved. Play with your teen even though you might take a pummeling. Listen as he explains the rules to you. Many games develop intellectual abilities, such as complex decision-making and problem-solving skills. He'll get to show you a world where he knows more than you do, and you'll get to appreciate his capabilities. When it's time to set limits, he'll respect your opinion because you're knowledgeable about the games and you've communicated that you care.

The MySpace Generation

Teenagers are growing up with a major influence in their lives that gives them more social power and public exposure than kids their age have ever had: online networking communities such as MySpace, Friendster, and Facebook.

If your adolescent daughter is too preoccupied to do her homework, it could be because she's updating her profile or responding to friend requests on one of these sites. If she's in tears, it's possible that a "popular" girl has just replaced your daughter in her "Top 8" or blocked her as a friend for the entire world to see (literally). And now she's got to concentrate on algebra and world history?

For generations, kids have survived the social cruelty of the junior high school years by staying under the radar. This choice is no longer available to your teen. In cyberspace, there's no place to hide, and there are no teachers, aides, or guidance counselors to protect young people.

Again, the best strategy for parents is to stay involved; but this can be tricky. Teenagers like their privacy when it comes to their friends. Psychologist and author Larry Rosen, PhD, is an expert in "techno-stress." In 2006, he found that:

- Only one-third of parents have seen their teen's MySpace page.
- Nearly half the parents claimed to have limits on their teen's MySpace use, but only 25 percent of the teens said those limits were upheld.
- Half the parents said that their teen uses the Internet from a location where the parent cannot supervise.

The challenge is to build trust and find ways to encourage your teen to share her experience with you. A MySpace page can be a source of pride and an exciting outlet for your teen's creativity. Keep a positive upbeat attitude. Don't use a tone that even hints of interrogation. If your teen feels like she's in a small room on a wooden chair under a single lightbulb, she will shut down, not open up. Help her feel emotionally safe—more like a picture of the two of you walking together, side-by-side.

Other Healthy Habits

Nutrition, exercise, supportive friends, freedom from clutter. . . The same behavior skills that help you keep a good, balanced brain chemistry for attention are even more essential for your child and his growing brain. Setting limits can be a challenge. No one wants to be "that parent"—the one with the carrots and celery sticks when it's your turn to bring snacks for the team. The key is balance.

Here are some tips to help you decide what limits to set:

- If you feel you're being pressured to say yes, buy some time. Tell your child, "I'll get back to you on that."
- Call on your observer self for some objectivity.
- Get more information—ask a teacher, a coach, a nutritionist, a doctor, or another parent whose opinion you respect.

Once you've made a good, solid, thoughtful decision, stick with it. Children need consistency.

Get Your Child to Make a Commitment

I once received a call from a dad who wanted to know how to get his son, Doug, to watch less television. After I heard the long list of things he had tried, I suggested that the three of us meet and come up with a plan.

First, Doug and his dad had to break their pattern of having control battles over TV. Doug's dad said that Doug was defiant. Doug said, "My dad doesn't own me."

In counseling, I asked them to take turns talking and listening. I asked the person who was talking to be brief and speak from the heart. And I asked the person who was listening to be quiet and truly listen, not just wait for his turn to talk again. I also asked the person who was listening to summarize what he'd just heard the other person say and reflect it back before he began his own response. I encouraged Doug and his dad to continue this practice of active listening at home.

Eventually, when he was no longer locked into having to prove a point to his dad, Doug had no problem admitting that TV "sucked him in." Doug's dad was floored by his son's insight. After awhile, Doug came up with this idea. Before he turned on the television, he would take a Post-it note and write down the time he planned to turn it off. He would put the Post-it note next to the screen so he would remember, even in his TV trance. The method worked. Interestingly, at our last session Doug proudly told me, "The TV doesn't own me."

Would the Post-it note method have worked if I had told Doug's dad to use it when he first called me on the phone? Of course not. There was no magic in this method, except for the fact that it was Doug's idea, so he was invested in it. Any reasonable method that *he chose* was the one that was going to work.

Nothing can replace taking the time to listen to children and help them develop their own tools for self-control. The more involved they are in planning their own success, the more likely they are to succeed. Here are some tips to help secure their commitment:

- Ask your child what he would do if he were the parent.
- Ask the empowering question: "By what time will you _____?"
- Give a "structured choice" that funnels your child into following the rules. Instead of saying, "Do your homework," say, "Would you like to start your history or your math?"

Step 5: Believe in Your Child

In today's competitive world every parent wants his child to have an edge. Prestigious private schools—even preschools—have long waiting lists. In school, after a full day of sitting still and staying focused, a kid doesn't get to run through the park pretending to be a galloping horse or a swooping eagle. Kids line up for language classes, computer classes, and ballet lessons.

In high school, building a strong college application is the equivalent of a full-time job. Kids take SAT prep classes with daily drills and practice tests. They take several advanced placement (AP) classes, write standout college essays, and join extracurricular activities to distinguish themselves.

If you're a parent, you wonder all the time: Am I doing enough? Is my child doing enough? Are other children doing more? Is my child falling behind? What more can I do? Will my child get into a good college?

If your child daydreams or gets distracted, you worry. While advances in children's diagnoses have brought help and hope to millions, parents today face another set of questions: Is my child just being a kid, or does he have a disorder? Is this a phase? Will my child grow out of it? Is this attention deficit disorder? Maybe it's a nonverbal learning disability? Should I get my child tested? Does he need special help? Will this go on his school records?

It's easier said than done; but for your child's sake, replace your worry with trust. If your child needs help, get it, but don't fret or obsess about it. Keep in mind that while you're dealing with your questions, your children are dealing with theirs: Am I smart enough? How come others can do that and I can't? Is there something wrong with me? Do I have what it takes? Will I get into college?

Your child's belief in himself starts with your belief in your child. Knowing you solidly believe in him protects your child when his own wolves of doubt howl and he needs the courage to carry on.

Spotlight Strengths

If your child is inattentive, particularly if he's been diagnosed with ADD, don't let his problems become his identity. This can happen inadvertently because getting the best help for your child is a time-intensive job and can take center stage without anyone's realizing it.

Recognize which skills your child needs to build so he can shore up his weaknesses; but make sure he identifies with his abilities, talents, and efforts. Stay aware of what you say to him and what you say about him to others. And set limits on what you say about him to yourself, particularly when you're at the end of your rope—a good time to reach for a change-of-state key.

The Number One Reason for Success

I chose "believe in the child" as step 5 because parents can continue practicing this step long after their children grow up and are on their own. But in importance, this step is actually number 1. It is the foundation for all the other steps.

In one study, successful adults who had struggled with attention problems as children were asked what had helped them most. Can you guess their answer? It was having one adult who believed in them.

14

The Power of Attention

If I have ever made any valuable discoveries, it has been owing more to patient attention than to any other talent.

—SIR ISAAC NEWTON

By now I hope you've chosen your favorite keys and put them on your own personal keychain. Joe, Meg, and Todd, whose stories you read in Chapter 2, chose their favorite keys. Here's how they used them to overcome their problems, and how they keep using them every day to succeed:

Logs on a Fire. Being an engineer, Joe liked the idea of learning more about the mechanics of his own brain chemistry. He immediately got the connection between adrenaline and his focus zone and wanted to know more. Once he understood that he'd pump more dopamine as soon as he finished a task, he put the information to good use. He'd say, "I need my 'finish juice.'" Joe continued to use self-talk and imagery to form new habits.

Joe compared all his new starts to kindling and his stick-to-it moods to logs. He imagined logs burning in a campfire and the good feeling of sitting there, cooking his dinner and knowing his fire will last as long as he needed it. In this way, he created the right mood for following through on his projects. He also liked the analogy of using a squirt of lighter fluid to get a fire going. It helped him to remember to stop squirting "new" and get on with the "do"—keywords that kept him in his zone.

These images helped strengthen Joe's observer self so much that he began to let himself see how his doughnuts and video games were really kindling, not logs. Once he did, he cut way back on them. No longer driven to game all night, Joe tried going to bed earlier. This proved to be a challenge, though. His mind raced and filled with worries and guilt about all the projects he should have completed by now. Joe realized that up to now, he had been playing video games until he was so tired he'd fall asleep right away, because subconsciously he feared lying in bed and having to deal with these unpleasant feelings. It took some time, but Joe practiced using keys from the anti-anxiety keychain to calm himself down and get to sleep.

A full night's sleep every night at the same time was a turning point for Joe. He found himself more in charge of his attention at work. In the mornings and at meetings he practiced asking the question "What am I *not* doing now?" And at home on weekends, he kept his metaphoric logs ablaze while he organized his computer desk and digital photos. He outsourced the wiring of his home entertainment center. No longer having such wide attention swings, Joe had enough new confidence in himself to make decisions like that.

Slow, Medium, Fast. Meg, the graphic artist, adopted a simple version of keeping track of her adrenaline score: she rated herself as slow, medium, or fast. She used her creativity to think of novel ways to add stimulation to her day with power breaks and mindful multitasking. She became a tea connoisseur, and even made her own blends of black, green, white, and herbal. And she put together various playlists of classical music, jazz, and dance rhythms from around the world. She found that listening to new music when she did her accounting helped her adrenaline score stay at "medium" for long stretches of time.

Meg liked having choices to psych herself up when she was "slow." Some days, she played salsa and drank spiced black tea. On other days, it was djembe drums with green tea and honey. What made the difference for Meg was realizing that she did have some control over her moods. Her confidence built as she saw that most times, with effort and strategy, she could get herself into her zone.

Meg used the keys from the procrastination-busters keychain to learn to meet deadlines at work. She used the sustainability keys to learn how to make a spreadsheet for her bookkeeping tasks. She packaged her lessons at the computer into small steps and built in rewarding breaks. For every twenty-minute Excel lesson she completed, she let herself spend ten minutes watching videos on YouTube.

One day, Meg searched for hours in her apartment for a piece of original artwork to show a potential new client. She knew it was there; she just didn't know where. That weekend, Meg decided it was time to tackle her clutter. At first, she could barely make herself do it. She realized she needed to be at her highest level of drive to begin to face the mess, so she made a plan. To get started, she waited for times when she was at a "high" rating on her adrenaline score, and then made cleaning up item 1 on her 3-item to-do list.

Also, Meg decided to ask some friends for help. Up till now, Meg might phone a friend and multitask if she was doing a mindless job such as folding laundry. But clearing her stacks of stuff was not a mindless job. She had to make decisions that required her attention. Meg had done many favors for her friends in the past, and she knew they wanted to support her. So she chose a few to confide in, and they became her phone buddies as she tackled piles of cards, notes, papers, magazines, and memorabilia. She treated herself to a Bluetooth earpiece to make it even easier to talk on the phone while she was sorting. Her friends turned the chore into a good-natured adventure, in their words, "in the name of feng shui."

Months later, when Meg's apartment was clutter-free, she began to notice that she spent more time at "medium" and "high" on her adrenaline score. With more space all around her, Meg felt less spacey herself.

I Am Not My Father. Todd started off using keys from the intensity-control keychain. Although none of his employees had ever brought it to his attention, Todd's own observer self kept him aware that he was short-tempered at work.

Todd's observer self also made him face his own role in his daughter's problems at school. Todd realized he had been pushing away his memories of himself at Becky's age. It was painful for Todd to remember how much he wished his dad had been there for him. "ADD," he thought, "stands for absent dad disorder."

Todd used the key of rescripting the past to heal from the sadness of his own lonely childhood. He also went to weekly counseling to sort through his feelings from the past. Todd used the goals-with-meaning keychain to decide to spend more time with his family in the evenings and on weekends. When he was tempted to go to the office or keep working on his laptop, the key he used was the deathbed test, to get back to his desire to be closer to his wife and children. He kept a copy of Steve Jobs's commencement speech in his desk drawer. Todd used self-talk to remind himself: "I am not my father."

Instead of taking his laptop to breakfast with the family, Todd stayed in his office and finished his work. At first he missed seeing the kids off to school. But by staying focused and efficient, he got more done and could then carve out time later in the day to give his family his undivided attention.

Todd promised to do something for Becky that he wished his dad had done for him: have one-on-one special time together. The question was: What could he and Becky do? Todd had no interest in going to the mall, and Becky was not keen on sports. It was Becky who first came up with the idea—could he teach her about the stock market? Online, they found a Web site where they each created a fantasy portfolio. They enjoyed competing to see who made more money, and they built a strong connection. Their time together gave Todd the chance to help Becky tone down her bossy ways. In addition, Todd and his wife began to give Becky less attention when she demanded it, and more attention when she was acting in a friendly and cooperative way.

Todd's father had died in his fifties of a heart attack, and Todd decided this was one more way he would not be like his dad. At his annual physical exam, Todd's physician talked with him about physical fitness. Todd had been getting some exercise here and there, but he decided to commit to a routine. Three times a week, Todd ran two miles. He was pleasantly surprised by how much this evened him out and helped his concentration on the job. Todd no longer felt so hyper or impatient all the time. He still kept his competitive edge, but he replaced his fear of loss with a vision of fulfilling his goals. Driven by desire, not fear, Todd now stays in his focus zone most of the time and sustains his motivation to succeed.

Are We Humans or Trained Seals?

Joe, Meg, and Todd used their new attention skills to bring out the best in themselves. In addition, Todd and his wife used their attention to reward Becky's cooperative behavior. When we use attention on purpose to influence another person's behavior, are we being manipulative?

Some people don't like the idea of using attention as a reward. They say it feels too calculating—as if they're treating a person as a lab rat instead of a human being. The fact is that we influence each other's behavior with our attention whether we realize it or not. When you're aware and intentional, at least you can deliberately choose which behaviors to support and which behaviors to discourage.

For several weeks, "What Shamu Taught Me About a Happy Marriage" (June 25, 2006) by Amy Sutherland remained the most frequently e-mailed article in the *New York Times*. At home, Sutherland had come to recognize that nagging her husband about minor annoyances only made matters worse. While she was writing a book about a school for trainers of exotic animals, a lightbulb went on in her head. She decided to try the same techniques as animal trainers on her husband, and she discovered that she got results. *She used her attention to reward behavior she liked and she ignored behavior she disliked.*

If her husband threw even one dirty shirt into the hamper, she thanked him. At the same time she ignored the soiled clothes on the floor, which to her pleasant surprise began to disappear. Sutherland explained that trainers call this technique "approximations," and that they reward each small step toward learning a new behavior.

When Sutherland's husband went storming around the house looking for his keys, she quietly said nothing, a technique called "least reinforcing syndrome" (LRS). He calmed down and called to her, "Found them."

Finally, Sutherland reported, she was complaining incessantly about her painful new braces and her husband was saying nothing. She realized that now he was giving her LRS—and, she reported, it worked.

Attention is a power like any other. It can be used for good or bad. You can use your attention to promote desirable behaviors or undesirable behaviors in yourself and others. Knowing what you're doing as you're doing it, gives you the chance to use your power wisely.

The Attention Economy

In 1971, Dr. Herbert Simon, who won the Nobel prize in economics, first observed, "A wealth of information creates a poverty of attention." In today's world, information is plentiful and attention is scarce. As a result, we live in a new "economy of attention" where attention is a rare and valuable currency.

In *The Attention Economy*, business experts Thomas Davenport and John Beck conclude that "understanding and managing attention is now the single most important determinant of business success." In the twenty-first century we face a lopsided case of supply and demand. Our most pressing problem is "not enough attention to meet the information demands of business and society."

In the *Economics of Attention*, Professor Richard Lanham of UCLA similarly observes that we are moving from an economy of things to an economy of attention. In our information-based world, what we are short of is the attention to make sense of all our information.

It can be helpful to think about attention as currency. When we do, we promote awareness of its value as an investment that brings us returns—depending on the choices we make every day.

If you were dealing in gold, you'd use a scale to weigh every ounce. When you complete a cash transaction, you count the money you hold in your hands. Attention is the same kind of resource. Every ounce of concentration counts. Learning to stay focused empowers you. It pays to remember that *your attention has worth*.

When you practice the skills you need to stay in your focus zone, you are rich in the currency of our attention economy. You hold the purse strings, so you can buy what you want from a treasure trove of knowledge unheard of just a generation ago. The vast wealth of the information age becomes yours, to learn, grow, discover, enjoy, and achieve your life goals.

Attention Is How We Create

In a few moments, when you finish reading this book, what will you focus on next? Work? Play? Family? Friends? Finances? Remember, *what you put your attention on grows*.

We can never be distraction-free; nor would we want to be. If you train yourself to ignore a laughing child, a fragrant rose, a simple kindness, a brilliant rainbow, or a glowing sunset, you will have fewer of these joys, not more. Centuries ago Socrates warned us, "Beware of the barrenness of a busy life."

Mary Lou Retton, the first gymnast outside eastern Europe to win the Olympic all-around title, said this about the 1984 Summer Olympics: "There can be distractors, but if you're isolated from the heart of the games, the Olympics become just another competition." The same is true of life itself.

It is my hope that you will take the keys you learned in this book to deliberately pay attention to what matters the most to you. The more you do, the more you will create the life you want for yourself and for the people you love.

APPENDIX

The Eight Keychains—
A Quick Guide

Keychain 1 ⚷ Self-Awareness

⚷ Your Observer Self

⚷ Your Adrenaline Score

⚷ The "What Am I *Not* Doing Now?" Question

Keychain 2 ⚷ Change of State

⚷ Four-Corner Breathing

⚷ Power Break

⚷ Mindful Multitasking

Keychain 3 ⚷ Procrastination Busters

⚷ Confidence Builders

⚷ Lighting the Fire

⚷ Rescripting the Past

Keychain 4 ⚷ Anti-Anxiety

⚷ Reality Check

⚷ Make a Plan

⚷ Thought Substitution

Keychain 5 ⌖ Intensity Control

- ⌖ Cooling Off
- ⌖ Uncover the Fear
- ⌖ Assertiveness Skills

Keychain 6 ⌖ Motivate Yourself

- ⌖ Goals with Meaning
- ⌖ Sustainability Tools
- ⌖ Deathbed Test

Keychain 7 ⌖ Stay on Track

- ⌖ Self-Talk
- ⌖ Attitude Shift
- ⌖ Mental Rehearsal

Keychain 8 ⌖ Healthy Habits

- ⌖ Lifestyles of the Calm and Focused
- ⌖ Supportive Friends
- ⌖ Living Clutter-Free

RESOURCES

Introduction

"How Much Information 2003?" was produced by the School of Information Management Systems at the University of California at Berkeley, and is available at www2.sims.berkeley.edu/research/projects/how-much-info-2003.

1: What Is Your Focus Zone?

The Yerkes-Dodson law was first published in R.M. Yerkes and J.D. Dodson, "The Relation of Strength of Stimulus to Rapidity of Habit-Formation," *Journal of Comparative Neurology and Psychology*, 18 (1909): 459–482.

On the state of flow, see Mihalyi Csikszentmihalyi's *Flow: The Psychology of Optimal Experience* (New York: Harper Perennial, 1991).

Step-by-step instructions for Jacobson's progressive muscle relaxation technique are at en.wikipedia.org/wiki/Progressive_relaxation.

2: Bored, Hyper, or Both?

On the inner game, see W. Timothy Gallwey's *The Inner Game of Tennis* (New York: Random House, 1997).

3: Attention in the Digital Age

Malcolm Gladwell explains rapid cognition and thin slicing in *Blink* (New York: Little, Brown and Company, 2005).

The analysis by the Parents Television Council of increased violence on TV is at www.parentstv.org/PTC/publications/reports/stateindustryviolence/main.asp.

4: What Are We Doing to Our Brains?

For a review of neuroplasticity studies, see Jeffrey M. Schwartz, MD, and Sharon Begley, *The Mind and the Brain* (New York: Harper-Collins, 2002).

On Richard Davidson's research of Tibetan monks' meditation, see John Geirland's "Buddha on the Brain," *Wired*, 14.02 (2006): www.wired.com/wired/archive/14.02/dalai.html. The study on western subjects, "Meditation Experience Is Associated with Increased Cortical Thickness," by Sara Lazar and her associates is at *NeuroReport*, 16, no. 17, November 28, 2005, www.neuroreport.com.

The brain science of multitasking is explained in Claudia Wallis's "GenM," *Time*, March 27, 2006: 48–55.

5: Emotional Skills

On emotional learning, see Daniel Goleman, *Emotional Intelligence: 10th Anniversary Edition* (New York: Bantam, 2005).

Your adrenaline score is based on the Subjective Units of Disturbance Scale (SUDS), introduced by Joseph Wolpe in *Psychotherapy by Reciprocal Inhibition* (Stanford, CA: Stanford University Press, 1958).

The study of children playing GameBoy while waiting for surgery was conducted by Anuradha Patel at the University of Medicine and Dentistry of New Jersey. See www.umdnj.edu/about/news_events/releases/04/r041210_gameboy.htm.

6: Confronting Fear and All Its Cousins

On procrastination, see Piers Steel, "The Nature of Procrastination," *Psychological Bulletin*, 133, no. 1 (2007): 65–94; and Jane Burka, *Procrastination: Why You Do It, What to Do about It* (New York: Da Capo Press, 2004).

7: Mental Skills

For Erik Erikson's developmental stages throughout the lifespan see en.wikipedia.org/wiki/Erik_Erikson.

A video of the 2005 Stanford University Commencement Address by Steve Jobs is available at www.youtube.com; a transcript can be found at www.stanford.edu. Each site has a search feature: enter "Steve Jobs Commencement."

8: Structure without Pressure

Research on recalling the names of supportive friends by James Shah was reported in "Automatic for the People: How Representations of Significant Others Implicitly Affect Goal Pursuit," *Journal of Personality and Social Psychology*, 84, no. 4 (2003): 661–681.

9: Behavior Skills

The study linking TV watching in toddlers and attention problems later in school, "Early Television Exposure and Subsequent Attentional Problems in Children" was conducted by Dimitri Christakis and published in *Pediatrics*, 113 (2004): 708–713. The recommendations of the American Academy of Pediatrics can be found at aappolicy.aappublications.org/cgi/content/full/pediatrics;107/2/423.

James Rosser's study demonstrating the benefits of videogames to train laparoscopic surgeons is described in Michel Marriott's "We Have to Operate, but Let's Play First," *New York Times*, February 24, 2005.

For more about Benson's relaxation technique, see Herbert Benson and Miriam Klipper, *The Relaxation Response* (New York: HarperTorch, 1976).

On people's attitudes toward risk, including a readable account of Kahneman and Tversky's prospect theory, loss aversion, and endowment and sunk cost effects, see Peter Bernstein's *Against the Gods: The Remarkable Story of Risk* (New York: Wiley, 1998).

10: Outsmarting Interruption and Overload

The classic study on personal control by Bruce Reim, David C. Glass, and Jerome E. Singer, "Behavioral Consequences of Exposure to Uncontrollable and Unpredictable Noise," was published in the *Journal of Applied Social Psychology*, 1, 1 (1971): 44–56.

On continuous partial attention, see www.lindastone.net.

For links to the studies on cognitive overload, see www.yourfocuszone.com.

11: Defeating Distraction in the 21st Century

On jet lag, see the MedlinePlus site, maintained by the U.S. National Library of Medicine and the National Institutes of Health, www.nlm.nih.gov/medlineplus/ency/article/002110.htm.

12: What If You (or Your Children) Have Attention Deficit Disorder?

A list of books and articles on learned helplessness is available at www.ppc.sas.upenn.edu/lh.htm.

The "Hunter in a Farmer's World" book is Thom Hartmann's *Attention Deficit Disorder: A Different Perception* (New York: Underwood Books, 1997). Yuan-Chun Ding and associates published "Evidence of Positive Selection Acting at the Human Dopamine Receptor D4 Gene Locus" in the *Proceedings of the National Academy of Science*, 99, no. 1 (2002): 309–314.

Edward M. Hallowell and John J. Ratey wrote *Driven to Distraction: Recognizing and Coping with Attention Deficit Disorder from Childhood Through Adulthood* (New York: Touchstone, 1995).

13: Teaching Kids to Pay Attention

Mirror neurons and learning through modeling are explained by Daniel Goleman in *Social Intelligence: The New Science of Human Relationships* (New York: Bantam, 2006).

For parents and teachers of children who struggle in traditional classrooms, see my first book, *Dreamers, Discoverers, and Dynamos: How to Help the Child Who Is Bright, Bored, and Having Problems in School*, formerly titled *The Edison Trait* (New York: Ballantine Books, 1999).

14: The Power of Attention

On the attention economy, see Thomas H. Davenport and John C. Beck, *The Attention Economy* (Boston: Harvard Business School Press, 2001); and Richard Lanham, *The Economics of Attention* (Chicago, University of Chicago Press, 2006).

For an up-to-date list of resources, including the Web sites listed here as active links, visit www.yourfocuszone.com

---

ACKNOWLEDGMENTS

This book is possible only because of the clients I've seen in my practice. Thank you for your courage, confidence, and resourcefulness. All of you are a part of this book: you taught me what works and what doesn't, what matters and what does not.

I'm grateful to my agent, Robert Shepard, for his confidence and support from the onset of this project. I appreciate his wise counsel, gentle strength, and impressive breadth of knowledge. I thank my editor, Leslie Meredith, for believing in the importance of this book, for her many helpful ideas and suggestions, and for the benefit of her expertise and guidance. My thanks to everyone at Free Press. Andrew Paulson, your can-do attitude is a joy.

My gratitude extends to my colleagues and friends for the honest, stimulating discussions that have contributed to this book. Sincerest thanks to Dave deBronkart for his originality, perceptiveness, and willingness to brainstorm whenever lightning struck. Dr. Mark Cooper, thank you for helping me simplify my scientific explanations without sacrificing accuracy. I am appreciative of the suggestions and support so warmly given by Marjorie Camp, Aline Christiansen, Lynn McBrien, Dr. Joel Oxman, Lori Oxman, Marcy Rogers, my parents John and Lucy Palladino, and my sister Maria Gill.

Three people have worked with me steadfastly from blank sheet to finished book. My mirror neurons and I are blessed beyond words that they are members of my own family. With all my heart, I thank my husband, Arthur Cormano, for his faith in me from the start. I appreciate his encouragement, dependability, and hard work, enthusiastically helping me with everything from manuscript suggestions to office equipment. Thank you, Arthur, for taking care of our daily needs so I could be in my focus zone and write. I am grateful to my daughter, Jennifer Cormano, for her unwavering support, incisive suggestions, and creative spirit. Thank you, Jen, for being an excellent sounding board and for helping me see points of view I might otherwise have overlooked.

Finally, I thank my daughter, Julia Cormano, who generously gave her time, attention, and considerable skill to this project from proposal to final draft. I am grateful to her for thoughtfully reading the manuscript chapter by chapter as I wrote it. Her versatility— from insightful advice to adept drawing of the illustrations— amazed me. Thank you, Julia, for understanding the value of this book, and for improving and strengthening its message every step of the way.

INDEX

(Abbreviations following page references: t=table, f=figure)

Index

Index

Index

Index

ABOUT THE AUTHOR

Lucy Jo Palladino, PhD, has gained recognition as one of the country's leading experts in attention. She is an award-winning psychologist with over thirty years of professional experience in this field.

Dr. Palladino has appeared on television, on radio, in newspapers, in magazines, and on the Internet. She's been featured in *Family Circle*, *Men's Health*, the *Los Angeles Times*, the *Washington Post*, the *Boston Globe*, and *Web MD*. She was the resident psychologist for the *Morning Show* on KFMB-TV, the CBS affiliate in San Diego, California.

In her practice, Dr. Palladino has seen people from all walks of life: executives, entrepreneurs, engineers, inventors, artists, designers, information technology workers, attorneys, athletes, and performers. She's worked with parents who juggle their roles inside and outside the home. She's counseled students and consulted with educators from kindergarten to postgraduate studies. She's taught psychological solutions and skills to thousands of people of all ages.

Dr. Palladino's extensive practical experience complements her impressive credentials in the field. In 1978, her doctoral dissertation, "Cognitive Strategies for Self-Control: The Use of Self-Instructions to Resist Distraction," was decades ahead of its time. Dr. Palladino was the principal investigator of a federal research grant. She has published articles in professional journals, has presented papers at national conferences, and was on the clinical faculty of the University of Arizona Medical School. In the 1980s, when Dr. Palladino saw the advances that elite athletes were making in attention control, she trained with an eight-time Olympic sports psychologist. She has cross-fertilized her clinical and consulting work with sports psychology techniques ever since.

Dr. Palladino is listed in the National Register of Psychology and serves on the Sports Psychology Committee of the San Diego Psychological Association. Since 1976, she's been a member of the American Psychological Association. She's also a long-standing member of Phi Beta Kappa who's retained a rigorous approach to the study of attention, while developing plain-language explanations and methods to help people solve everyday problems. Her commitment to excellence plus her warmth and humor makes her a well-liked, highly respected, and entertaining speaker and workshop leader.

When Dr. Palladino wrote her first book, *Dreamers, Discoverers, and Dynamos: How to Help the Child Who Is Bright, Bored, and Having Problems in School* (formerly titled *The Edison Trait*), *Publishers Weekly* observed, "Parents and educators alike will find this compelling reading." It went on to win the San Diego Book Award and the San Diego Press Club Journalism Award, and to be named an Editor's Choice and one of the top three parenting books of the year at Amazon.

Dr. Palladino's Web site is www.lucyjopalladino.com.